THE
COMPLETE
ALLERGY
BOOK

JUNE ENGEL, PHD
WITH ISOLDE PRINCE

FIREFLY BOOKS

A FIREFLY BOOK

Cataloguing in Publication Data

Engel, June
        The complete allergy book

ISBN 1-55209-203-8

1. Allergy – Popular works. I. Title.

RC584.E54   1998   616.97   C97-932379-7

Published in the United States in 1998
by Firefly Books (U.S.) Inc.
P.O. Box 1338
Ellicot Station
Buffalo, New York, USA
14205

Diagrams: Lianne Friesen
Electronic formatting: Heidy Lawrance Associates

Printed and bound in Canada

98 99 00 01 6 5 4 3 2 1

Contents

Acknowledgments

In preparing this book I have been immeasurably helped
by many experts involved in allergies and their management, including geneticists, allergists, immunologists,
dermatologists, pediatricians, respirologists, biologists, psy-
chiatrists, social workers, ophthalmologists, family physicians
and emergency medicine specialists – from coast to coast across
the North American continent. Some of them have checked
and rechecked specific chapters of the book several times over
– and to them I am especially grateful.

First and foremost, I would like to thank the many people
who encouraged me to write on this complex subject, and
the many specialists I met and interviewed at innumerable
clinics and at conferences, who directly or indirectly helped
with the book.

I am immensely indebted to Dr. Gordon Sussman, who carefully checked and revised the entire book. In addition, I owe
very special thanks to Dr. Karen Binkley, Dr. Desmond
Colohan, Dr. Stanley Epstein, Dr. Milton Gold and Dr. Peter
Vadas for checking and rechecking various chapters, patiently
steering me in the right direction. I am equally grateful to
Dr. Allan Becker, Dr. Bernice Krafchik, Dr. Susan Tarlo and
Dr. Barry Zimmerman, for meticulously reviewing several sections of the book, sometimes twice over. I must also make
special mention of Dr. Zave Chad and other members of the

Canadian Society of Allergy and Clinical Immunology for their support.

For further help with specific sections or chapters, I must thank Dr. Brian Barber, Dr. Irv Broder, Dr. Ken Chapman, Dr. Isser Dubinsky, Dr. Pierre Ernst, Dr. Stephen Feanny, Dr. Bernard Fresco, Dr. Mitchell Friedlaender, Dr. David Golden, Violetta Jovanovic, Barbara Klich, Dr. Aubert Lavoie, Dr. Eric Leith, Dr. Arthur Leznoff, Dr. James Martin, Dr. Jonathan Matz, Dr. Ricky Schachter, Dr. Robert Schellenberg, Dr. Allan Slomovic, Dr. Susan Swiggum, Dr. Wendy Tamminen, Dr. Peter Thomas, Dr. Richard Warrington and Dr. Elizabeth Weber.

I must also express my gratitude to Agriculture Canada, the Ontario Lung Association and Metro Toronto Lung Association, the Allergy/Asthma Information Association, the Ontario Society of Allergy, Asthma and Immunology, and the Canadian Society of Allergy and Clinical Immunology for their prompt replies to my endless queries.

Last, but far from least, I owe thanks to my assistant, Madeline Koch of Wordcraft Services, and to my researcher, Isolde Prince, without whom the book would never have been finished.

Introduction

Allergies, which affect an estimated 40 million people in North America alone, are a major reason for doctor visits and absences from school and work, and cause untold distress. This book is intended to help all allergy sufferers, and those caring for them, understand the disorder and manage it as effectively as possible, in partnership with competent healthcare providers.

We speak of "allergy" as if it were one disorder, but with its multitude of symptoms and its numerous triggers it seems more like many. It's hardly surprising that early medical writers failed to recognize the connection between someone who sniffles and sneezes every spring, someone whose lips swell on eating fish and someone who goes into shock and dies from a wasp sting. Even modern allergists sometimes have a hard time classifying allergies, since they can be categorized according to their triggers, the parts of the body they affect or the age at which they usually occur.

I have tried to organize this book in a simple, understandable manner, to give you accurate, up-to-date, in-depth knowledge that will help you "take charge" and deal with your problem – whether it's seasonal or year-round; whether it's triggered by a food, pollen, insect or drug; whether it affects your skin, eyes or lungs. My emphasis is on how you can improve your lifestyle and environmental control to reduce your symptoms, and how, when necessary, you can make use of medications, with the aid and advice of medical experts.

Although the description of what goes wrong in allergies, in Chapter Two, is somewhat complicated, it is intended to give you some understanding of the many complex immune-system changes that cause allergic reactions, and to explain why and how present and future treatments may work. Chapter Five includes detailed lists of anti-allergy medications currently available, describing which types suit particular allergies, to help you make the right choices, and use these drugs to best effect. Some common brand names are included as examples, but this is in no way an endorsement; your pharmacist or physician can help you decide between products.

Although children's allergies are often similar to those of adults, some aspects are quite different. Chapter Eight focuses on the specific problems of allergic children.

Over the last few decades, scientists have made considerable strides in diagnosing and treating allergies. Today, more than 90 percent of those with hay fever and year-round allergic rhinitis can ease their symptoms effectively; eye symptoms can now be relieved more readily and safely; and many asthma sufferers can control their disease using a greater variety of anti-inflammatory medications. New guidelines are improving the emergency care for severe allergic reactions.

Immunotherapy – allergy shots, among the oldest allergy therapies, at one time inappropriately and unscientifically dispensed – has been much refined. Purified extracts for immunotherapy are being developed, and scientific studies have identified those for whom allergy injections provide appropriate and effective treatment with little risk.

Scientists have also made major advances in understanding the biochemical steps in the allergic process, and new drugs and therapies based on this research are being developed. For example, vaccines that prevent or block allergic reactions are now in the testing phase in the U.S. and Canada, and may soon be on the market.

However, despite all this progress, many concerns remain – especially the apparent increase in allergies, with the accompanying misery, missed work days and rare but often needless fatalities. The rising incidence and severity of asthma, especially among the young, are particularly worrisome; the increase is attributed largely to failure to recognize asthma and treat it early, and to the fact that asthma's severity is often underestimated until it reaches life-threatening proportions. Chapter Nine gives a thorough explanation of the mechanism and triggers of asthma, a rundown of new treatment approaches, practical tips for day-to-day management and ways to develop an "action plan" to help keep severe attacks at bay.

I hope the information in this book will allow you to understand what causes your allergy, and to develop the most effective management strategies possible – founded on knowledge and *evidence-based* methods, rather than hearsay or "hit and miss" therapies. It should also help you communicate better with your medical caregivers, and know which questions to ask to get as much relief as possible.

J.E.

ONE

Overview

Allergies are noncontagious reactions in which people begin to itch, sneeze, wheeze, swell up, break out in hives (red, raised welts), have difficulty breathing or occasionally collapse, in response to normally harmless substances or conditions. Allergies are among the most frequent and distressing health complaints, even though many of those afflicted don't seek medical help. They are thought to affect 40 million people in North America alone and, tragically, about 500 Americans and 50 Canadians die each year from their allergies, often through failure to get the right treatment in time. But while allergies can be life-threatening, they are mostly known for the inconvenience, misery and health-harming complications they cause – for the distress, the many absences from school and work and the billions of dollars spent annually in North America on treatments, some appropriate, others useless. In some cases, people spend money on treatments that may even worsen the condition.

Medical experts have long been puzzled by the curious fact that some individuals develop serious symptoms, and a few even die, from agents that don't trouble most people. Those prone to allergies are said to be *atopic* or "hypersensitive" to certain triggers. ("Atopic" means "out of place.") A tendency to allergic disorders or *atopy* often runs in families. But allergies can also arise for no identifiable reason.

The allergy-producing substances – called *allergens* – can be inhaled (as with pollens, dust and molds), ingested (as with foods), injected (as with insect venoms, vaccines and some medications) or absorbed through the skin (as with some plant products and cosmetics). The answers to why some people develop allergic symptoms from the presence of a cat, a few inhaled pollen grains or a taste of peanuts, while most people remain unaffected, are now being uncovered as scientists discover why and how allergies make people miserable.

Allergy Reactions Follow Repeated Exposure

An allergic reaction is brought on by exposure to specific foreign substances, or allergens – mostly proteins, or small molecules attached to proteins – that sensitize the body's immune system so that it reacts to normally harmless substances as though they were dangerous intruders. Contrary to popular misconception, allergy attacks don't usually begin out of the blue. It generally takes a period of "sensitization" through one or more exposures to a specific trigger (or triggers) to build up an allergic response. When someone first wears latex gloves, for instance, or when a cat first joins a household, there is usually no reaction, but repeated contact may eventually cause a latex rash or a cat-induced runny nose and itchy eyes. Once someone is sensitized, it may take only tiny amounts of the allergen – traces of cat dander or latex rubber – to trigger symptoms, sometimes severe ones.

Occasionally someone appears to have an allergic reaction on first encountering a food or other allergen, but there must have been unknown exposure on some past occasion. Sometimes it takes long-term exposure – months to a year or more – to build up an allergy, for instance to certain pollens, as in hay fever.

Considering the vast number of foreign substances we encounter each day, it's surprising how few provoke allergies. For example, of all the foods eaten, only a few commonly cause allergies in North America – in particular, cow's milk, eggs, fish, shellfish, legumes (such as peanuts and soy) and tree nuts. Similarly, of all the different types of pollen that fly about in North America, hay fever is commonly caused by those from only a few grass, weed and tree species. Depending on their entry route, allergens cause different symptoms. Inhaled allergens such as pollen and molds typically cause nasal and lung symptoms; those eaten (ingested) may produce tongue tingling, gastric upsets and swollen breathing passages. Ingested and injected allergens tend to induce the most severe, body-wide reactions.

The extent and severity of an allergic response range from the merely annoying to the life-endangering. For example, the stuffy nose and runny eyes of hay fever, and the contact rash that develops from some cosmetics, are distressing but not life-threatening, although they can lead to complications, especially if left untreated. In contrast, a food allergy or bee sting that jeopardizes breathing or affects the heart and circulation can culminate in allergic shock, and even in the death of an otherwise healthy person. *Anaphylaxis*, the most severe allergic reaction, affects several body systems at once and can occur within minutes. Its possible warning signs include widespread hives, flushing, a sudden drop in blood pressure and difficulty breathing. It can be rapidly fatal if not immediately treated. (See Chapter Three.)

The Historical Perspective
Adverse reactions to wasp stings and certain foods were among

the first allergies reported. In the fourth century B.C. the Greek physician Hippocrates observed that milk made some people sick to their stomachs and gave them red skin weals. A few other foods – such as shellfish and nuts – seemed to cause similar symptoms, and occasionally made people go into shock. Another Greek physician, Galen, noted that some plants, such as poison ivy, caused skin reactions in certain individuals. Hippocrates and other early medical men tried to explain these unpredictable responses in terms of toxins that somehow harmed just a few people. Several centuries later, the Roman philosopher Lucretius, in his scientific poem "De Rerum Natura," observed: "What is food to some may be bitter poison to others" – or, as the saying now goes, "One man's meat is another man's poison."

In the sixteenth century, the Italian physician Leonardo Botallo remarked on a patient who got headaches and began to sneeze on smelling roses; another Italian physician reported someone who became ill whenever a cat was in the room; and an Italian astrologer cured an archbishop's asthma by removing his featherbed and feather pillows. In the mid-1800s, the condition we now call hay fever was traced to grass and weed pollens. Later, scientists showed that tiny amounts of pollen from specific plants could bring on nasal stuffiness, sneezing and eye irritation. The condition was worst during the pollination season, when pollen counts were high. In the late 1800s, a German dermatologist, Josef Jodassohn, invented the "patch test" to show which substances, if put on the skin, would trigger itchy, red patches, revealing themselves as allergy provokers. He also showed that dust mites – tiny sightless creatures, distantly related to spiders, that live in dust – would often cause an allergic rash and nasal stuffiness.

Why is shock serious?

The medical term "shock" refers to inadequate circulation of blood to the body's tissues. Shock can be caused by a loss of blood (hemorrhagic shock from severe bleeding), by a severe infection (septic shock) or by numerous other factors. Allergic shock is caused when the blood vessels become "leaky" and dilate (widen) so that the pressure of circulating blood ("blood pressure") drops.

Since blood carries oxygen and essential nutrients to the cells of the body, a drop in blood pressure can disrupt the body's functions. A person "in shock" will tend to be pale and cool, and may be dizzy or may pass out. If shock is not treated, it can cause death.

The word "allergy," which comes from the Greek *allos* or "other" and *ergon* or "work," was coined in 1906 by the Viennese pediatrician Clemens von Pirquet. The term captures an essential aspect of allergy – namely, that it "alters" the "work" (reaction) in an allergic person's body.

In 1910 Sir Henry Dale, a British scientist, identified *histamine* – a substance released by our body tissues, but first isolated from fungi, rye and other plants – as a key "mediator" in the body's allergic response. He showed that histamine acts to make smooth muscles contract, thus narrowing the breathing passages, and to make blood vessels dilate, thus lowering the pressure of the blood, also causing inflammation and pruritis (itching). This explained some aspects of the allergic reaction: the hives, itching, swelling and in worse cases the breathing problems due to congested airways. Once histamine was identified as a key agent responsible for some allergic symptoms, the search began for antidotes – forerunners of today's widely used *antihistamines*.

Allergies Today

There are no exact figures for the number of people who suffer from allergies, as many do not consult physicians; they just medicate themselves or cope with the discomfort. However, one or more allergies are thought to affect 15 to 20 percent of North Americans. According to the U.S. National Institutes of Health (NIH), one in five Americans has an allergy-related illness during his or her lifetime. Statistics from the Canadian Society of Allergy and Clinical Immunology show that about one in six Canadians is treated each year for an allergic disorder, including seasonal hay fever, asthma, eczema, hives, and cat, food, insect and drug allergies. One in five North American children sees a physician because of an allergy, and some children are hospitalized for it.

In particular:
- An estimated 15 to 20 percent of North Americans suffer from hay fever along with nasal symptoms triggered by pollens, dust, animal dander (a mixture of dried saliva and skin flakes) and other airborne particles.
- About 1 to 3 percent of infants are allergic to cow's milk proteins.
- About one in 600 allergy-prone people is at risk of severe anaphylaxis (a life-threatening reaction).
- About 5 to 10 percent of the North American population have asthma, with one in seven children affected, and over half the asthma cases are allergy-related. The incidence of asthma has increased by 33 percent during the past decade, with deaths doubled since the 1980s – especially among children.
- Some 1 to 2 percent of North Americans have food allergies.
- Generally, allergy-prone people – for example, those who suffer from hay fever or dust allergy – are not more vulnerable to insect stings, or drug or food allergies. However, people with asthma who also have allergies are at above-average risk of severe reactions.

- About 3 percent of the adult North American population have an insect-venom allergy, with an estimated 25 to 50 insect-sting deaths annually.
- About 1 to 3 percent of North Americans have a drug allergy, and 5 percent of these may be allergic to more than one medication. Penicillin and its relatives are the medications chiefly responsible for severe drug allergies; almost 10 percent of penicillin-treated patients are at some risk.

Allergies and the Immune System

An allergic reaction is an overreaction of the body's immune system. The immune system is part of the defense mechanisms that protect the body against harmful foreign ("non-self") substances that enter or threaten it. The immune system signals white blood cells to rush to the "attack site" and engulf the invading particles, and also produces antibodies that inactivate or destroy specific invaders. Unlike a normal immune reaction, which is launched against dangerous bacteria, viruses or parasites, an allergic reaction is a misguided attack against inoffensive proteins such as those in cat dander, pollens, dust mites or food. Although it has been known since the early 1900s that allergies are due to immune-system activity, only in the late 1960s did researchers finally identify the specific "allergy antibody" – *immunoglobulin E*, or *IgE* for short – responsible for some allergic reactions. Today we know that although IgE antibodies are involved in some types of allergy, others may be caused by different immune-system components (see Chapter Two).

As the biochemical processes involved in the allergic response are unraveled, scientists understand better how to develop drugs and therapies against them. Besides antihistamines, which block the action of histamine, newer medications are being designed to block other mediators and other steps in the allergic reaction.

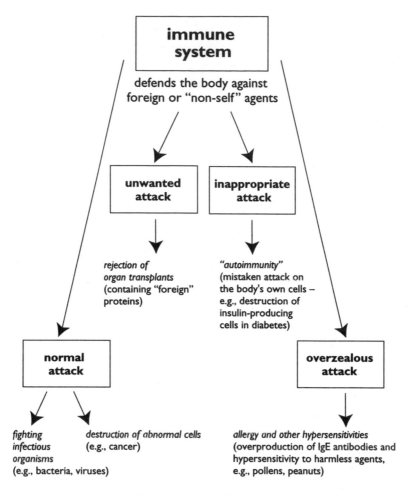

The Immune System

Identifying Allergic Triggers

A thorough and careful medical history, together with appropriate tests, can usually identify an allergy. The medical history – with details about the onset, duration and type of symptoms

– is key in tracing the cause. The allergist will ask about the home, school and work environments, and about diet and lifestyle. Skin tests (and occasionally blood tests) may be done, using extracts of the suspected allergen(s) to determine whether the complaints are really due to an allergy and, if so, what triggers the reaction. In skin tests a tiny amount of diluted allergen extract is put under the skin, through a prick or scratch, to check if there's any reaction. A red, raised hive-like eruption appearing in 15 to 20 minutes is a "positive" test, indicating possible allergy to the substance. Skin tests should always be done by physicians trained in immunology and allergy in case of severe reactions. They should *never* be done in a setting without full emergency backup.

Common Allergy Triggers
Inhaled allergens
- pollens (grass, tree, weed)
- dust mites
- animal proteins (from saliva, skin or urine)
- mold spores
- insect parts

Injected allergens
- insect venoms
- medications
- vaccines
- hormones (e.g., insulin)

Ingested allergens
- foods
- drugs taken by mouth

The basics of the "allergic cascade"

An allergic reaction occurs because the immune system has become sensitized to a particular allergen. Once it "knows" its supposed enemy, the immune system reacts immediately against it. In some cases, specific antibodies are produced to inactivate the invader. But whereas most antibodies (IgG, IgM, IgA, IgD) are protective – helping to fight harmful bacteria, viruses, fungi and other toxic substances – the IgE antibodies involved in allergic reactions are produced against harmless substances. (In "non-IgE-mediated" allergies, different components of the immune system react to the allergen.)

In IgE-activated allergies, the IgE antibodies bind to and activate special *basophils* in blood and *mast cells* in the linings of the nose, throat, lungs, eyes, skin and digestive tract, making them release allergic "mediators." These potent chemicals mediate (produce) the manifestations of allergy – the itching, skin reddening, hives or rash, runny nose, wheezing, tissue swelling and inflammation. Different allergic mediators produce different effects. Some increase blood-vessel "leakiness," allowing fluids to escape into surrounding tissues, leading to swelling and congestion. Others constrict the lungs' airways, producing asthmatic wheezing and other breathing problems. As well, mucus-producing cells secrete fluid in an attempt to wash away the offending allergen, producing a runny nose and watery eyes. All these reactions contribute to the immediate reaction or so-called allergic cascade that occurs upon contact with a foreign agent. If they are very severe, the combined body-wide reactions can produce an extremely serious allergic reaction called *anaphylaxis*, which can be life-threatening.

Besides the immediate reaction, a more recently recognized *late phase*, or delayed reaction, often develops several hours later. The result can be a second wave of swelling and inflammation, or a return of the anaphylactic attack.

Absorbed (contact) allergens

- plant components
- latex
- dyes
- fabric chemicals, paints, pesticides, resins
- metals (e.g., nickel in jewelry)
- cosmetic ingredients, nail polish, hair dyes, fragrances

Birth of Allergic Reaction

Allergen
enters body,

causes white
blood cell to
produce IgE
antibodies,

white
blood cell

Allergen
re-enters body,

antibodies

allergen bonds
to IgE antibodies
on mast cell,

antibodies
attach to
mast cell.

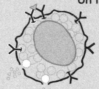

mast cell
releases various
mediators including
histamine.

Who's Most Likely to Get Allergies?

Among the general North American population, 15 to 20 percent have a known allergy. Although the tendency to be allergic may be inherited, the specific symptoms and the allergens to which someone reacts are quite individual. For example, Emily has had severe asthma since childhood; in the summer she develops hay fever, and she is also allergic to certain fruits such as melons, which give her a tingly sensation inside her mouth. Her mother was allergic to horses, and would get wheezy and breathless when she went horseback riding. Emily's five-year-old daughter, Bernie, has a severe cat allergy with nasal symptoms and has had a tendency to eczema since she was a baby.

Most allergic people are afflicted with only one or two specific allergies. Others have multiple allergies, perhaps to several airborne triggers such as pollen, fungal spores, animal dander and dust mites. An unlucky few suffer from allergies affecting many parts of the body, triggered by a variety of allergens. The degree to which a person's immune system responds to any given antigen is partly under genetic control. Studies show that two allergic parents have about a 70 percent chance of producing an allergy-prone child. The odds decrease to 30 percent if only one parent has allergies and to 10 percent if neither has any allergies.

Allergic people may inherit an above-normal number of mast cells, or may be genetically primed to respond to allergens and produce IgE rather than the usual antibodies. Although genetic factors increase the chances, heredity isn't the whole story. Even with no family history of allergy, one person in ten develops one or more allergies. Studies of genetically identical twins show that even though one twin is allergy-prone, there's a 40 percent chance that the other twin won't have allergies, as nongenetic factors also play a role.

Key qualities of allergens

- *Chemical make-up*: Allergens are small molecules. Most are proteins, but some are *haptens*, chemicals able to bind with proteins. The hapten-protein combination triggers the response.

- *Ease of access to the body's immune system*: Tree and grass pollens, for example, are light and float high in the air, where they can be breathed in, whereas most flower pollens are heavier and fall to the ground, where they are less readily inhaled. Grass, ragweed or tree (often maple and birch) pollen is more allergenic than marigold, rose or tulip pollen.

- *Size of particles*: Most allergens are small enough to penetrate the mucous membranes (linings) and cause sensitization. Pollen particles may lodge on the surface of mucous membranes in the nose and eyes, causing symptoms, but smaller particles such as cat dander may be more deeply inhaled and can trigger more widespread symptoms. The allergen in cat dander (a mixture of dried saliva and skin flakes) is composed of tiny particles measuring 0.05 to 20 micrometers, which can get deep into the breathing passages, triggering severe nasal congestion and lung inflammation in susceptible people. Its tiny size means that it is easily airborne and can be suspended in the air for as long as three to six months after the cat has gone.

- *"Allergenicity"*: It's not clear why some substances are more allergenic than others. Peanut proteins, for example, are highly potent and can provoke severe, lifelong allergies.

- *Frequency of exposure*: The more commonly an allergen is encountered, the more likely it is to trigger an allergy. Ragweed allergy, for instance, is common in many parts of North America – no surprise as one square mile (2.6 square kilometers) of ragweed reportedly produces 16 tons of pollen per season. In North America many infants are allergic to cow's milk and eggs; in Japan, where rice is a staple infant food, many children are allergic to rice; in Sweden, where fish is common fare, many are allergic to fish.

- *Level of exposure*: Exposure itself does not always provide sensitization; sometimes a certain level of exposure must be reached. Workers who breathe in a lot of flour dust, or are often exposed to latex particles, are at increased risk of allergy.

Different Allergic Disorders Hit Different Folks

- *Hay fever (seasonal allergic rhinitis)* – meaning inflammation in the nose – is produced when IgE antibodies made by the immune system activate mast cells, causing symptoms in the upper respiratory tract. It's triggered by specific pollens from grasses, weeds or trees appearing in spring, summer or fall. Each pollen-producing plant has its own seasonal pollination peak. Springtime allergies may be due to ash, birch and elm, among others; midsummer pollen allergies are often due to grasses such as orchard, rye and bluegrasses. Fall allergies may arise from ragweed and other weed pollens. Chief symptoms are sore, red, watering eyes, a stuffy, itchy nose, endless sneezing, a clear nasal discharge, blocked sinuses, perhaps earache, and itching of the roof of the mouth and/or ears.

- *Non-seasonal or perennial (year-round) allergic rhinitis* – with nasal stuffiness, sneezing, watery eyes and a perpetually sore or burning throat – is also an IgE-mediated reaction, and is triggered mainly by indoor allergens such as dust mites, cockroach parts, mold or fungal spores and cat or dog dander.

- *Eye (ocular) allergy, or allergic conjunctivitis* – with eye redness, itching and swelling, perhaps a sticky discharge – frequently accompanies hay fever, or is precipitated by direct contact with a cosmetic or other substance.

- *Urticaria (hives)* – with red, itchy, raised welts on any part of the skin, and some swelling – may be triggered by a food, insect sting, drug, or local contact (e.g., with latex or a dye), or can be a sign of anaphylaxis, so it must be taken seriously. If the hives affect deeper tissues there may be considerable swelling. Hives can be "acute" – coming on suddenly, lasting a short while and then disappearing; or "chronic" – persistent and long-lasting. Chronic hives, frustratingly, often have no traceable cause and may not be due to an allergy.

- *Food allergies* – IgE-mediated reactions, sometimes serious – are most commonly due to cow's milk, eggs, fish, shellfish, nuts, legumes (such as peanuts or soy), and occasionally certain fruits and vegetables. A food allergy is typically heralded by tingling, burning and swelling of the tongue and lips, nausea, stomach cramps, diarrhea, perhaps throat swelling and difficulty breathing. The symptoms can extend to the whole body and be rapidly life-threatening. (See Chapters Three and Eleven.)

- *Animal allergies* – especially to cats and dogs – are increasing with the rising popularity of household pets. Veterinarians and laboratory personnel may become sensitive to other animals, and farm workers may develop horse allergy. The response typically includes a stuffy, itchy nose, sneezing, red, sore, weepy eyes, wheezing and hives.

- *Insect allergies* can be severe, and are mostly triggered by venom from the sting of certain *Hymenoptera* (bees, wasps, yellow jackets, hornets), and also by some biting insects. There may be a large, inflamed swelling at the attack site, perhaps becoming more widespread, with hives, throat swelling, weakness and shock, requiring immediate medical treatment. However, a systemic (total-body) insect-sting reaction can occur even with negligible swelling or soreness at the attack site.

- *Drug and vaccine allergies* – sometimes severe – are most frequently triggered by antibiotics (such as penicillin and sulfa drugs), anesthetics, heparin, dextran, ASA (aspirin) and certain radiocontrast dyes (used in X-ray imaging).

- *Atopic dermatitis (eczema)* – characterized by an angry, itching, scaly, weepy skin rash – is quite common in young children and can be linked to an allergy. Skin tests may identify a trigger, but in about one-third of cases no obvious cause is found.

- *Contact dermatitis* – not an IgE-mediated response but a different immune-system reaction, with an itchy skin rash or hives – is set off by repeated contact with numerous triggers such as a plant chemical, metal, cosmetic or manufactured product. It can be very disabling and may even force people to change jobs. (See Chapter Twelve.)
- *Asthma* – a noncontagious lung disorder, sometimes triggered by allergies – involves coughing, wheezing (a whistling sound on breathing out), shortness of breath, airway inflammation and mucus collection in the lungs' bronchial passages which can seriously impair breathing.

Are Allergies Increasing?

Allergic disorders are thought to have become more common in North America and Europe during the last 15 to 20 years, and researchers are trying to determine the reasons. In particular, the incidence of the "allergic triad" – rhinitis, asthma and nasal polyps – has almost doubled in many countries since the 1970s. One survey of allergies among Welsh children found that between 1973 and 1988 the number with hay fever rose from 9 to 15 percent; the number with asthma increased from 6 to 12 percent and the number suffering from eczema rose from 5 to 16 percent.

Other studies record a doubling of the numbers of U.S. children admitted to hospital with asthma since the 1970s. Not only hospitalizations but also deaths from asthma have been increasing. In the U.S., for example, more than 5,000 asthma deaths were reported in 1991, a number more than twice that for 1977 – with no clear reason. Death rates from this condition have also risen in Europe, Australia and other developed nations. (See Chapter Nine.)

The "allergic march"

Athough allergy can strike at any age, a first allergic episode frequently appears before the age of five, and the condition may disappear with increasing age. For example, atopic dermatitis (eczema) almost always makes its first appearance in infancy or early childhood, and resolves as the child gets older. Cow's-milk protein allergy, also common in infancy, tends to vanish as the baby's immune system matures. While some allergies, particularly food allergies, often persist into the teen and adult years, few of the elderly still sneeze their way through the hay-fever season.

Sometimes allergies change as children mature, with one group of symptoms being replaced by another in a characteristic pattern called the "allergic march." Early food sensitivities may be replaced by sensitivity to airborne allergens (*aeroallergens*), causing nasal and lung problems. For example, as an infant Jenny suffered from eczema all over her face. The eczema disappeared by the time she was about a year and a half, only to be replaced by hives and vomiting immediately after she ate eggs. These symptoms resolved a couple of years later, but Jenny went on to develop hay fever in her teens. Her hay fever may well lessen in later life, so she will have fewer symptoms.

Epidemiologists, who study the distribution and causes of diseases, believe that some of the reported surge in allergic disease is only *apparent*, reflecting greater public and media interest. Allergy awareness is a fairly recent phenomenon and, together with the greater likelihood of accurate diagnosis, may partly explain the apparent rise. As one woman, now a senior, puts it: "When I was a child I used to get attacks of a sniffly thing, with sneezes and coldlike symptoms. I would just go to bed for a few days. Today I would probably be diagnosed as allergic, but then we wouldn't have thought of allergy or even gone to a doctor. We knew about hay fever and asthma, and we'd heard some horror stories of people dying from insect bites, but that was about it; we just wouldn't think of allergy as an explanation for what was wrong with us."

Air Pollution: One Suspected Reason

While the seeming increase in allergies may reflect greater media publicity, more public interest and better diagnosis, many experts suggest that there is probably a real rise in allergy incidence as well. The reason isn't known, but air pollution (especially vehicle and diesel fumes) and other environmental changes may aggravate allergic symptoms. Epidemiological evidence linking air pollution with an increase in allergy comes from Japan, where hay fever was almost unknown before World War II but is now common. It's mainly triggered by tree pollens, so if hay fever were merely a matter of breathing in cedar and other tree pollen it would probably be most prevalent in rural areas. However, hay fever is far more widespread in Japanese cities, near highways, suggesting that there are city air components that increase vulnerability. Allergic disease is also generally more prevalent in developed areas such as Europe and North America than in underdeveloped areas, suggesting that there may be something about the modern urban lifestyle that promotes it.

Another proposed explanation for the rise in allergic disease is the "tight building theory." According to this concept, today's energy-efficient urban buildings, with their sealed windows, have created the perfect microclimate for accumulating allergens such as dust mites, animal dander, fungal (mold) spores and insect parts. Supporters of this theory point out that many of us spend much time indoors, breathing in allergens, which exacerbates our respiratory allergies. Other possible allergy-inducing aspects of our Western lifestyle include the rising popularity of pets, and changes in dietary patterns – for example, less breastfeeding, and earlier introduction of cow's milk and solid foods that can sensitize an infant's immune system.

Commercial products may also play a role. The frequency

of allergic reactions is directly related to the number of people exposed ("population exposure") to a given allergen. For example, exposure to latex, a natural product from trees used in surgical gloves and medical devices, has spawned an ever-growing crop of latex allergies. When new consumer items or drugs appear on the market, product allergies often develop. Once penicillin became readily available after World War II, the frequency of allergic reactions to this medication jumped, until today penicillin is one of the most frequent causes of severe anaphylactic shock. Similarly, the increasing diversity of peanut products, their presence in many prepared foods, their growing popularity as snack items – particularly for young children – and their presence in restaurant meals is producing what some call an epidemic of peanut allergies.

Approaches to Allergy Treatment

There are three main ways to manage an allergy: remove or avoid the provocative agent; quench or prevent the reaction with medications (pharmacotherapy); or, for selected allergies, try immunotherapy, "desensitization" using allergy shots with specific allergen extracts. In addition, people can try to prevent allergies from developing, by taking certain precautions – especially avoiding known triggers and reducing stress. Researchers have shown that, although emotional tension and stress may aggravate allergic conditions, they are not the primary causes.

Avoiding Known Allergen(s)

The first and best treatment for allergies is avoidance – steering clear of the triggering agent(s) as far as possible. That may mean not eating eggs, fish, peanuts or other food allergens, trying to keep pollens and molds out of the home, making the house as dust-free as possible, getting rid of a pet (or at least banning it from the bedroom) or avoiding allergy-provoking cosmetics, latex or other items.

Pharmacotherapy

Many medications are now available to help prevent attacks and relieve symptoms, used separately or in combination.

- *antihistamines* – there is a wide range to choose from, the newer ones being less sedating – used as tablets, syrups, sprays or eyedrops
- *mast-cell stabilizers* – such as cromolyn (also called "cromoglycate") – used as eyedrops or a nasal spray to help prevent attacks
- *corticosteroids* – used either topically, as a spray, or by mouth – to mute the inflammatory response

Immunotherapy

"Desensitizing" allergy injections are suitable for selected allergy cases. Better-purified allergen extracts, and new guidelines for their use, are improving the success of immunotherapy. Provided the *right* allergen(s) are used, in *high enough* concentrations, the technique may help desensitize people allergic to insect-sting venoms, identifiable seasonal pollens, animal dander and possibly dust mites.

Preventing Allergies

Indoor allergen levels can be reduced by keeping homes free of dust and mold, and avoiding pets. Women from known allergic families, whose children are at high risk of developing allergies, can breastfeed their babies for at least six months, delay the introduction of solid foods, and start infants on non-allergenic foods (avoiding cow's milk, eggs, seafood, nuts and peanuts) for perhaps the first two to three years, or even longer.

Be Wary of Unconventional Tests and Therapies

Despite the fact that allergies are recognizable immune-system reactions, the mistaken notion continues to circulate that many or most inexplicable discomforts or vague health complaints are due to some "allergy." In their search for relief, ever more people blame multiple environmental factors and turn to "alternative" or unconventional therapies outside standard medical practice. These unconventional treatments – often based on traditional oriental methods – include homeopathy, naturopathy, herbalism, hypnosis, massage therapy, acupuncture, therapeutic touch and some risky practices such as coffee enemas.

If you're tempted to try alternative methods, remember that they have usually not been evaluated by standard scientific methods, and have not been clinically *proven* effective or safe.

Standard medical practice refers to "evidence-based" methods of diagnosis and therapy, based on scientific principles. Alternative or nonconventional methods of testing and treatment, although not scientifically proven safe and effective, may suit and help some people – provided they do no harm. However, check out their merits and validity before trying them.

For example, "neutralization therapy" – which combines wide-ranging environmental avoidance and elimination diets with the use of vitamin and mineral supplements and certain salts to "neutralize" the body's allergies – has been shown by scientific studies to improve only 4 percent of those who try it. Of the others, 44 percent remained unchanged and 52 percent found symptoms worsened.

In general, conventional medical caregivers have a wary attitude to alternative therapies, although some are beginning to endorse their use as "complementary" therapy – alongside conventional treatment, but not instead of it – provided they do no harm. Spurred by popular interest in unorthodox therapies, many physicians now promote certain nonconventional methods in addition to traditional medical treatment. The Office of Alternative Medicine, established by the U.S. National Institutes of Health, is examining their validity and usefulness.

However, it's wise to thoroughly check out any unorthodox therapy you're considering, and to discuss it with your physician, in case it could conflict with or undermine medical treatments you are receiving. Some alternative methods are of no proven value; some may be downright harmful. Some clinical ecologists and certain environmentalists who call themselves "allergy therapists" may trade on mistaken ideas about allergy to propagate and publicize various tests and "cures" of doubtful value, some of them very time-consuming and expensive. Being cautious in using such procedures may be a good idea. The American Academy of Allergy, Asthma and Immunology has issued statements saying that the concept of clinical ecology is an "unproven methodology" and that people considering such treatment should recognize its "experimental nature."

During the 1980s, a popular concept of "total allergy syndrome," or sensitivity to multiple environmental agents – first dubbed "twentieth-century disease" but now called "multiple chemical sensitivity"(MCS) – led to many so-called allergy or clinical ecology treatments for a syndrome not yet proven to be either allergic or total. Those hit by this incapacitating syndrome believed themselves "allergic" to a vast range of triggers and products, from electromagnetic fields and automobile exhaust to paint, perfume, adhesives, furnishings, carpet glue, detergents, numerous plants, food additives, cigarette smoke and virtually any item with a distinct odor. People afflicted by MCS did (and still do) experience profound distress from minute amounts of the incriminated chemicals – well below threshold levels that bother most people. Many blamed the workplace for their ills.

Failing to obtain satisfactory medical treatment, MCS sufferers often seek help from clinical ecologists and self-proclaimed specialists in environmental medicine – sometimes traveling to distant clinics and undergoing costly therapies of unproven usefulness. Some are advised to drink only triply distilled water, administer sublingual (under-the-tongue) "neutralizing drops" at the onset of symptoms and isolate themselves in "environmentally safe" havens within their homes. In many cases they withdraw from society entirely and spend most of their time at home, admitting only a few select visitors "free of all scents and pollutants."

Although people with MCS frequently see themselves as victims of multiple chemical allergies, their complaints – headaches, poor concentration, thought aberrations, abdominal distention, stomach upsets, throat tightness (although the throat looks normal) and an inability to get air into the chest (but no wheezing) – lack the hallmarks of real allergic (immunological) reactions. "The majority of people with multiple chemical sensitivity," says one allergist, "have no evidence of environmental allergy – no elevation in IgE levels, no sign of increased mast-cell mediators (histamine, cytokines or leukotrienes), or other signs of immune-system changes. Their symptoms are vague and nonspecific."

Some researchers have theorized that MCS could arise in certain people from nutrient deficiencies, or through proximity of the brain's limbic system to the olfactory (smell) lobe. (The brain's limbic system is the seat of human emotions and urges – anger, love, sadness, sexual drive, self-preservation and survival.) Whether there is any truth to these theories remains to be seen. In any case, MCS sufferers need to reduce their exposure to irritating volatile odors and organic solvents, and many benefit from counseling, nonjudgmental psychotherapy, support and stress-management advice.

Anyone considering unconventional tests or cures should try to distinguish fact from fiction, remembering that allergies arise from definable, distinct immune-system activity with a recognizable set of symptoms. Many allergists and immunologists warn people to beware of self-styled "clinical ecologists" claiming they can identify allergic triggers by unvalidated tests such as hair analysis, "skin titration" (measurement), feeling the pulse, injection of the sufferer's own urine or "cytotoxic" (white-blood-cell) tests. The result of misguided trust could be a long course of unproven (and perhaps expensive) therapy, false hopes and failure to get correct diagnosis and suitable treatment. Alongside medical therapy, many unconventional therapies work well, but anyone considering their use should discuss the pros and cons with a medical caregiver.

TWO

Understanding Allergies: What Goes Wrong

An allergic reaction is an inappropriate immune-system response that causes symptoms in a certain subset of the population. *Specificity* is the hallmark of all immune responses: people are usually allergic to only a few specific substances. For example, someone sensitive only to the allergen found in red cedar dust will react on inhaling this tree compound, not others; those sensitive only to the protein in cat dander will respond to that, not to animals in general; those allergic only to certain shellfish will react on eating those varieties but not others; and so on. Thus, although many people say they're "allergic" to something because they feel it has some vague effect on them, the allergic response is *not* vague; it's a definite, identifiable immune-system activity triggered by a particular foreign agent that's harmless to most people.

Although the material in this chapter is complex, knowing how the immune system produces allergic symptoms can help you control it. It can also help you understand the many new approaches that are under scientific study.

Where Does the Allergic Response Come From?

The allergic response results from the immune system's remarkable ability to distinguish "self" from "non-self" substances, and its ceaseless attempt to fend off agents that are "non-self," which are termed *antigens*.

The body's immune defenses are gradually built up from birth onwards, as we encounter more and more environmental agents. Every second of the day our bodies face an onslaught of bacteria, viruses and other potentially harmful microorganisms and chemicals. These tiny, unseen attackers are first warded off by the body's front-line defenses, such as the skin. Those that manage to get past these defenses and enter the body, through breaks in the skin or by penetrating mucous membranes in the nose, throat, gut, or urinary or genital tract, are attacked by the immune system with a complex array of weapons that destroy invading intruders so they cannot make us ill or kill us. Blood rushes to the site, bearing white blood cells that engulf or destroy the foreign intruders; antibodies made by lymphocytes (special white cells) help to inactivate specific invading antigens.

Some lymphocytes have an inbuilt "memory," so that once a harmful antigen has been fought off, the immune system is "tagged" to recognize its re-entry and rapidly destroy it in the future, should it ever again penetrate the body.

Unlike most antigens, which are potentially dangerous, the distinguishing feature of allergens (allergy triggers) is that they are substances harmless to most people. Many allergens are commonplace proteins in foods, plants or animals, and the immune-system response to these innocuous substances that takes place in allergy-prone people amounts to overkill. IgE antibodies are inappropriately manufactured against harmless agents such as pollens, animal dander, or even nutritious staples such as peanuts, eggs and milk.

The IgE antibodies bind to mast cells in the mucous (lining) layers, and to basophils in the blood, stimulating them to "degranulate" and release powerful *vasoactive* mediators. ("Vasoactive" comes from the Latin *vas*, or "vessel.") The mediators – histamine, leukotrienes and a host of others – make blood vessels dilate and become "leaky," producing swelling and the all-too-familiar signs of allergy – the itching, rash, hives, weepy eyes, sneezing, nasal discharge, inflammation and other discomforts. In severe cases, respiratory failure, allergic shock and death may occur.

Why should so irritating, useless and health-harming an immune-system response have evolved? Scientists surmise that allergies may be part of the evolutionary development of the body's immune defenses mounted against parasites that were once rampant. In other words, the body's exaggerated immune response may be a throwback to the days when it was a valuable defense against widespread and harmful parasites such as intestinal worms and insect larvae – parasites that now no longer exist in most places. (Such immune-system reactions do still occur when the body needs to clear itself of parasites.) However, scientists do not yet fully understand why some people mount an attack against innocuous substances as though they were parasites, while most do not.

Unraveling the Immune System's Complexity

The immune system's key components are:

- *leukocytes* – special white blood cells (*leukos* is Greek for "white," and "cyte" means "cell") that include monocytes, macrophages, eosinophils, neutrophils and basophils, as well as lymphocytes (see below). Some rush to the attack site and engulf invading particles; others have other roles; and some play a part in allergic reactions. Although they are called "white blood cells," many mature in organs such as the thymus and lymph nodes;

- *lymphocytes* – white blood cells that play a key part in allergic reactions. They originate in stem cells in bone marrow, and then mature into "B" and "T" varieties. The *B-lymphocytes* (or B-cells) mature in the bone marrow, while those destined to become *T-lymphocytes* (or T-cells) leave the bone marrow and mature within the thymus gland. B-cells and T-cells have different roles in the allergic response.
  - *B-lymphocytes* make antibodies (immunoglobulins) that can inactivate specific antigens (foreign invaders). Any given B-cell can make one of five different antibodies: IgA (immunoglobulin A), IgD, IgG, IgE or IgM.
  - *T-lymphocytes* are divided into various classes and include cytotoxic (cell-killing) cells – which can recognize and destroy abnormal cells hit by infection or cancer – and "helper" cells. The *T-helper* cells are further subdivided into *TH1* and *TH2* types, depending on the chemical messengers they produce. TH1-helper cells make *interferon*, a substance (cytokine) with some antimicrobial properties. TH2-helper cells are allergy-aggravators, which make different *cytokines* (chemical signals) that stimulate B-cells to make IgE antibodies;
- *antibodies* made by B-lymphocytes, which inactivate or destroy antigens;
- *mediators* – such as *histamine, bradykinin, tryptase, leukotrienes* and *platelet-activating-factor (PAF)* – made and released by basophils in the blood and mast cells in the lining layers of the skin, nasal passages, eyes, mouth, throat, respiratory tract and gut.

Lymphocytes Play a Key Role

Lymphocytes of various types are strategically situated wherever foreign materials enter the body – under the skin and in the membranes that line the mouth, nose, eyes, intestines, and respiratory and reproductive tracts. Foreign agents that get past these lining tissues and penetrate deeper may be carried into lymph channels and then to lymphocyte-rich *lymph nodes*, where they are destroyed. (When lymph nodes are fighting infection, they can become noticeably enlarged as "swollen glands" in the neck or groin.) Invading antigens that get into the bloodstream are generally destroyed by lymphocytes in the spleen.

Some lymphocytes are short-lived and die soon after eliminating the antigen; others become long-living "memory" cells that divide into identical "daughter" cells to provide a dormant army ready to spring into action against a specific antigen. This means that if there is a subsequent invasion by that antigen, the immune system will be ready to supply a "secondary" response that is faster and stronger than the original immune reaction. (This is the basis of vaccination – a weak primary response to the vaccine leaves the body prepared for a strong secondary response in case the actual disease-causing agents have to be resisted.)

In an allergic response, both B- and T-lymphocytes play major roles. In IgE-mediated allergies – those triggered by IgE antibodies – the B-cells make the IgE antibodies, in response to a chemical signal (a cytokine) produced by the TH2-helper cells. Supposedly, the allergy-prone have more TH2-helper cells than non-allergic people. In non-allergic people, harmless foreign substances such as ragweed and bee venom trigger production of various antibodies that uneventfully clear the antigen without causing noticeable symptoms. But in allergy-prone people, the same innocuous agents provoke the production of IgE antibodies that stimulate mast cells to release the mediators that produce allergic distress. Although the mechanism isn't yet understood, the number of TH2 cells is

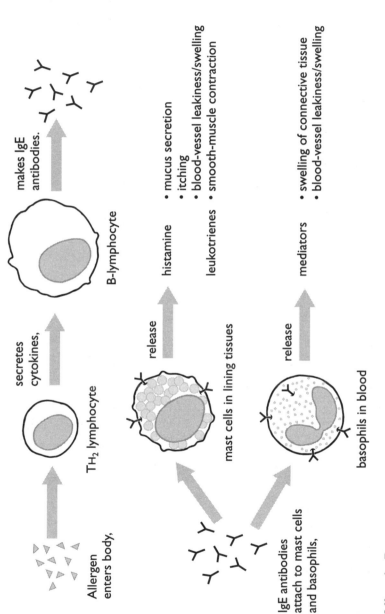

Allergic Process

thought to be under genetic control, explaining why people may inherit an allergic predisposition. Intense research is underway to find drugs that might turn off the allergy-producing action of TH2-helper cells, thereby halting the allergic cascade.

Four Basic Types of Hypersensitivity

The four main types of allergy are labeled I, II, III and IV, but also have descriptive names.

Type I, or IgE-mediated, Allergic Hypersensitivity

Type I hypersensitivity, or "immediate onset" allergy, develops in stages on repeated exposure to a specific allergen such as dust-mite feces, animal dander, foods, pollens, drugs and insect parts. The first encounter sensitizes the body and stimulates B-cells to produce IgE antibodies specific to the invading allergen. The IgE then binds to the surfaces of mast cells in mucous membranes and to basophils in blood. The mast cells and basophils may remain sensitized with IgE on their surfaces for many months, or even years. If the same allergen again enters the body, it is hooked onto the waiting IgE antibodies, making the mast cells and basophils "degranulate" – the medical term for the explosive discharge of mediators from their granules. The mediators, each with a different action, produce the allergic symptoms – the itching, puffiness, flushing, congestion, hives and other discomforts.

Once someone is sensitized, a type I or IgE-mediated allergy – as the name "immediate-onset" implies – usually surfaces within minutes or seconds of exposure to the allergen. The first symptoms to appear vary according to the type of allergen and the site of entry.

One of the mediators, histamine, is a key player in the early stages. In fact, histamine alone can cause much of the initial allergic impact. Many of the characteristic signs and symptoms of allergy can be mimicked by giving histamine infusions to animals, and can be blocked by antihistamines. Itchiness occurs when histamine stimulates nerve endings. Histamine and other substances relax smooth muscle around blood vessels. At the same time, both histamine and leukotrienes make the lining of blood vessels contract, enlarging the gaps between cells, so that fluid leaks out into surrounding tissues, causing swelling and inflammation. Mediators can also make airway muscles contract, leading to wheezing and difficulty breathing, or they can act on the digestive tract, causing nausea and diarrhea.

In the case of rhinoconjunctivitis (nasal and eye inflammation), airborne allergens such as ragweed pollen interact with IgE antibodies on mast cells in the linings of the nose and eyes, causing fluid leakage and increased mucus secretion. Likewise, the touch of an allergen may activate mast cells in the skin, causing blood-vessel expansion and leakiness, with consequent swelling and hives.

Allergens that are absorbed into the bloodstream can travel to sites far from the point of entry, causing more severe allergic symptoms all over the body; this is most common with drug, insect-venom and food allergies. For example, when a food allergen enters the body it activates mast cells all along the digestive tract, from mouth to intestines, leading to swelling and tingling of the lips, mouth and throat. Sudden smooth-muscle contraction of the intestines can cause nausea, vomiting and diarrhea. The allergen may also trigger blood-vessel dilation throughout the body, with a dramatic drop in blood pressure, and allergic shock. Activation of mast cells in the airways may produce constriction and asphyxiation (choking). So many changes all at once, in so many systems, can lead to anaphylaxis, a severe, systemic (multisystem) reaction that's potentially fatal. Such cases need immediate epinephrine (adrenalin) injection.

Type II and III Antibody-mediated, Non-IgE Hypersensitivity

While type I allergy is triggered by IgE antibodies, type II and type III allergies involve other immune-system components. In a healthy immune response, foreign antigens are cleared by one of several mechanisms. A little damage to bystander cells is inevitable. But type II and III allergic reactions may, for unknown reasons, actually work against the body. Otherwise healthy tissues can become targets of destruction by an antibody attack. Part of the body's organs or tissues may be altered, perhaps leading to *autoimmune* diseases such as rheumatoid arthritis, lupus erythematosus and some thyroid diseases. Diabetes mellitus results when the antibody attack destroys the insulin-producing cells of the pancreas. Similarly misplaced attacks may play a role in multiple sclerosis.

Type II, or antibody-mediated cytotoxic hypersensitivity, is often directed against foreign antigens lodged in or on the body's cells. For example, small molecules such as antibiotics can become absorbed onto the red blood cells, triggering antibody action against the drug. The antibodies may bind to the blood cells and destroy them, resulting in hemolytic anemia. In *Goodpasture's syndrome*, antibodies are directed against the kidneys and lungs, leading to kidney damage and lung disease.

Type III hypersensitivity, or immune-complex-mediated hypersensitivity, involves antibody-antigen complexes that are too large to be engulfed and destroyed by leukocytes, and are deposited in tissues where they stimulate destructive inflammation. If these complexes enter the blood, they can lodge in narrow passages and filtration sites such as the lungs, kidney, joints, arteries and skin, causing great damage and resulting in autoimmune diseases such as rheumatoid arthritis. The air sacs of the lungs (alveoli) can become hugely inflamed in this way, causing *extrinsic allergic alveolitis*, a type III hypersensitivity sometimes experienced by farmers, vets or animal fanciers.

Type IV, Delayed Hypersensitivity (DTH)

The first signs of type IV hypersensitivity usually appear 24 to 72 hours after exposure to an allergen, as opposed to the seconds or minutes taken for a type I allergy to appear. Type IV reactions often result from exposure to antigens such as nickel, cosmetic ingredients, poison ivy, latex additives and formaldehyde. The characteristic itching, rash, redness and swelling surface two to three days after contact. These reactions involve special immune-system T-cells found in the skin and lungs.

Once the triggering antigen is removed, the reaction slowly fades and the skin eruptions vanish. However, type IV allergies can be most uncomfortable and unsightly, and if the sites become infected they can lead to serious complications. If the eruptions are chronic or lingering, they can cause scarring and *granulomas* (internal scar tissue and bumps) near or at the affected site. Therapy for delayed hypersensitivity is avoidance of triggers and relief of the inflammation, usually with corticosteroids. Drugs that suppress the immune system, such as cyclosporin, are also occasionally used for severe cases.

THREE

Anaphylaxis: The Most Severe Response

naphylaxis, a term coined in 1902, means "excessive protection," and refers to the most severe of allergic reactions. Anaphylaxis is a generalized allergic response that affects many body systems simultaneously. Death may occur in minutes unless there is immediate treatment.

The allergens most liable to trigger anaphylaxis are drugs such as penicillin and some other antibiotics, insect venoms and foods. While anaphylaxis can swiftly kill, not all anaphylactic reactions are fatal. Nonetheless, anyone who has ever experienced a severe, body-wide allergic reaction must be on guard and take precautions.

The origins of anaphylaxis were first explored in the 1920s, when horse serum – used to make vaccine for diphtheria, scarlet fever, tetanus and tuberculosis – was found to induce fatal allergic shock. Since then, it's become clear that severe allergic reactions do not usually occur the first time someone encounters a foreign allergen, but only after the person has been sensitized (perhaps unknowingly) to a particular substance. In a few instances – especially in children – an anaphylactic attack seemingly occurs on the first exposure to a food or drug, but in such cases it's assumed the child was unwittingly sensitized – perhaps during breastfeeding, by substances the mother ate, or perhaps by hidden ingredients in a food or product.

What Exactly Happens in Anaphylaxis?

In essence, anaphylaxis is a *systemic* allergic reaction affecting many parts and systems of the body at once; it is the culmination of many immune-system events. As potent allergic mediators are discharged, they have a dramatic impact all over the body. Widespread, itchy hives may erupt on the skin, and perhaps also a spreading flush (redness and sense of warmth). Along the respiratory passages and in the lungs, the mediators produce swelling and congestion which can constrict the airways and hinder breathing. In the mouth and digestive tract, the mediators can make the tongue, lips and throat tingle and swell up. Sudden smooth-muscle contractions may produce nausea, vomiting and diarrhea. In the circulatory system, the mediators may trigger blood-vessel leakiness and expansion causing a dramatic drop in blood pressure, and perhaps also heartbeat irregularities. So many serious, even life-threatening events occurring all at once can kill within minutes, through heart failure or breathing problems.

The exact pattern of anaphylaxis varies from person to

A note on terminology

The medication used to treat – and perhaps save the lives of – people who suffer anaphylactic reactions is epinephrine, also known as adrenalin. This substance immediately counteracts the dangerous effects of anaphylaxis: it widens constricted airways, stops blood-vessel leakiness (raising blood pressure) and speeds up the heartbeat. Extracted from animal sources, or made synthetically, epinephrine resembles the hormone adrenalin made by our adrenal glands. Sometimes the terms "adrenalin" and "epinephrine" are used interchangeably.

How common is anaphylaxis?

We don't know exactly how often anaphylaxis occurs, or how many people die of it, but the condition is thought to be under-reported. The annual recorded incidence in the U.S. is about 3.2 cases per 100,000 people, or 8,000 cases a year, with 0.4 to 0.5 fatalities per million people per year – about 500 deaths a year, mainly from allergies to drugs, insect stings and certain foods. Statistics from the Canadian Allergy/Asthma Information Association show a proportional number of deaths in Canada from similar causes.

Deaths from anaphylaxis may occur away from home or far from medical aid, perhaps because someone fails to recognize the crisis and doesn't use (or delays using) life-saving measures, or has forgotten or neglected to carry an emergency injection kit. Experts believe that allergies may be responsible for more deaths than statistics reveal; the signs of a fatal allergic reaction (the skin weals, swollen throat and flushing) fade fast, so the sudden death may be wrongly attributed to a heart attack or other event. "Since anaphylaxis is largely under-recognized, under-treated and under-prevented," notes one allergist, "estimated numbers are probably on the low side, the number of reported fatalities likely being just the tip of the iceberg."

person, but once someone has had an identified anaphylactic reaction to a certain allergen – be it a drug, insect venom, certain food or other agent – the next time the same trigger is encountered there will likely be a similar reaction. While anaphylactic reactions are frightening and some are potentially fatal, most cases do not end in death. On the whole, the severity of anaphylaxis does not worsen from episode to episode, but this is not a foolproof rule. With time, if there is an extended period between anaphylactic attacks and re-exposure to the same allergen, the risk and severity of the reaction may fade, but this *cannot* be relied upon. For safety's sake, one must assume the worst – that the reaction could be severe – and act accordingly.

Recognizing Anaphylaxis in Time Is Vital

Regardless of the trigger, the signs and symptoms of anaphylaxis are usually similar. The tissues and systems most affected are those rich in mast cells – the skin, lungs, tongue, throat, respiratory tract, blood vessels and digestive system. Symptoms usually surface within minutes – sometimes within seconds – of swallowing, being injected with or (occasionally) inhaling the allergen. The key warning signs are a rash or hives, itching, flushing, tingling ("pins and needles"), tongue swelling or burning, throat swelling, anxiety, faintness and a racing pulse.

More than 80 percent of those afflicted develop widespread hives and swelling during an attack; 70 percent have upper and lower respiratory tract symptoms and wheezing or breathing trouble; 25 percent have a drop in blood pressure with accompanying dizziness or lightheadedness. But not all allergic symptoms necessarily occur in all people on all occasions. Some people can hardly breathe but have no obvious heart irregularities; or heart failure can occur without obvious breathing problems.

Quite often, people who experience an anaphylactic episode have no idea what it was or why it happened, and don't bother to follow up. They may brush it off as a fluke, leaving themselves open to an equally or more dangerous reaction next time around. Recognizing the reaction and knowing what to do about it aren't always easy, unless you have already experienced an attack, know what it is and what causes it, and can warn others of your allergy and how to treat it.

If the problem is recognized and properly explained to the person, repeat occurrences can often be prevented. "No one who's had an anaphylactic episode," notes one emergency-department chief, "should leave the emergency unit without receiving some information about the condition, guidance for follow-up, referral to an allergist for a thorough assessment, and instructions for emergency action."

Common Warning Signs of Anaphylaxis
Any combination of the following:
- hives (red, raised skin weals)
- itching (of armpits, groin, or any part of the body)
- swelling (of throat, tongue, or any body part)
- throat tightness or closing
- difficulty swallowing
- wheezing
- difficulty breathing
- red, watery eyes
- runny nose, sneezing
- face flushing
- vomiting, diarrhea, stomach cramps
- changed voice
- altered color
- dizziness
- irregular heartbeat
- anxiety
- sense of impending doom
- drop in blood pressure
- fainting or prolonged unconsciousness

Note: All or some symptoms can occur at the same time.

Managing Anaphylaxis

Injection of epinephrine is the immediate treatment for anaphylaxis, and the usual dose is 0.3 mg for adults, 0.15 mg for
children under 33 pounds (15 kilos) in weight. It may be vital
to administer the shot well before a hospital or physician can
be reached. "Speedy injection is paramount," notes one expert.
"Failure to use it promptly is more dangerous than using it
improperly." Bystanders may give the injection from an emergency kit to someone collapsing from allergic shock if the

person has asked them to do so. (The injection can be given *through* the fabric of pants or a skirt, although heavy outdoor clothing may have to be removed.)

Side-effects of the injection are pallor, a tremor or shakiness and a rapid pulse; these pose little danger except to someone with a heart condition. In children and young people, serious side-effects such as cardiac disturbances and hypertensive (high-blood-pressure) crises are extremely rare, and the life-saving benefit of epinephrine for suspected anaphylaxis outweighs any small risk of adverse effects.

People who have an anaphylactic attack must *always* get medical attention, even if the emergency injection seems to have cleared the symptoms. All cases should be taken to an emergency department at once. Emergency-room personnel may administer oxygen (to help protect the heart and brain), and may give intravenous fluids to counteract shock and raise blood pressure. They may also give corticosteroids to relieve inflammation, and antihistamines as backup therapy – *never* to replace epinephrine. (Antihistamines combat only one mediator – histamine – whereas epinephrine reverses the action of many mediators.) Besides an H_1 histamine-blocker (such as diphenhydramine), which blocks histamine at a number of sites, an H_2 blocker (such as ranitidine), which blocks it in the gut and intestines, may also be given, especially if there are widespread and resistant hives.

Occasionally, people in anaphylactic shock are rushed to a cardiac or trauma unit and the anaphylaxis goes unrecognized, so no epinephrine is given. "It is crucial for people with anaphylaxis to receive an *immediate* injection of epinephrine," notes one Toronto expert in emergency medicine, "not other drugs such as antihistamines or steroids – which may be backup measures but not first-line therapy. It is a mistake to think that one can just keep an eye on things and act if they worsen, or to hope the reaction won't happen."

"Late Phase" After-Effects

Even though the immediate signs of anaphylaxis may fade quickly on treatment with epinephrine, there is always a risk of a second, equally life-endangering "late phase" anaphylactic event occurring within 3 to 12 hours of the first, requiring more epinephrine. (If the second wave follows hard on the heels of the first, it may just appear to be prolonged anaphylaxis.) Corticosteroids such as prednisone may be given, as well as oxygen, bronchodilators to open the airways, fluid replacement to raise blood pressure, blood-pressure-elevating medication and other support measures.

"It is critical that those caring for people with anaphylaxis keep them under observation," warns one emergency-medicine expert, "as a late or delayed reaction can occur, usually within 6 to 8 hours." One study found a recurrence in 20 percent of cases. Therefore, people should be kept under surveillance for 12 hours after an initially severe reaction seems to have cleared. (They may be detained for less time after a milder reaction.) "It is equally important after someone has been treated for anaphylaxis," adds the expert, "not to let him or her leave the emergency unit without knowing the dangers of a repeat occurrence and being told what to do."

Identifying the Causes of Anaphylaxis

Investigating an attack of anaphylaxis can take lots of detective work, because the cause may be far from obvious. Anaphylaxis can be mistaken for fainting ("vasovagal syncope"), a more familiar but usually harmless event. Fainting is managed by simply helping the person lie down.

Penicillin is the most frequent drug cause of anaphylaxis. It is closely followed by cephalosporin (another antibiotic). Insect stings are the next most frequent cause – in particular the venom of the *Hymenoptera* class, which includes bees, wasps,

Anaphylactoid or "pseudoallergic" reactions

Distinguishing anaphylactic reactions from others that seem similar can be tricky. *Anaphylactoid* reactions closely mimic anaphylaxis, and are equally dangerous, and occur mostly in response to medications and physical triggers such as sunlight, heat and intense cold. However, anaphylactoid reactions are *not* mediated by IgE antibodies but *directly* stimulate the release of allergy-provoking mediators such as histamine from mast cells. Drugs such as ASA (called "aspirin" in the U.S.) and other non-steroidal anti-inflammatories (NSAIDs), opiates and gamma globulin, dialysis membranes and radiocontrast material (used in X-ray imaging) typically cause such pseudoallergic reactions. They require the same treatment as anaphylaxis: immediate epinephrine injection. (See Chapter Fourteen.)

yellow jackets and hornets – followed by foods as the next most frequent cause. The head of one emergency department notes that those rushed in with anaphylaxis from food are most often people allergic to peanuts and seafood. "About 40 to 50 percent anaphylax from food allergies," he says, "and the rest from a variety of triggers, particularly insect stings, penicillin and vaccines, or they are set off by skin prick tests or allergy shots with a provocative allergen."

No one should have allergy tests or injections in any location without full emergency backup. "It's essential," notes one allergist, "to have life-saving aids on hand when doing allergy tests or giving allergy shots. People must be observed for a minimum of 20 minutes after an allergen injection, to make sure no adverse reactions occur – watching for signs such as flushing, swelling or itchiness."

But that doesn't mean allergy tests should be avoided. The director of an anaphylaxis clinic notes that "one big favor you can do for someone who has experienced allergic shock is to help identify its cause, so the precipitant can be avoided. Someone who doesn't know what to avoid can suffer anaphylaxis at any time."

Who Is Most at Risk?

Roughly 1 percent of the North American population is at risk of anaphylaxis. Near-fatal or fatal anaphylactic episodes are most common among adults, although children may be at as great, or greater, risk because of their inability to recognize and act on the emergency. In children, anaphylactic episodes tend to produce fewer cardiovascular (blood system and heart) problems and more airway obstruction, swelling and hives.

People who are taking beta-blocker drugs for high blood pressure or other disorders are at increased risk of anaphylaxis, because they will not respond to epinephrine injected as an antidote. If you have experienced allergic reactions, you may be advised to use other drugs instead of beta blockers.

Living with the Risk of Anaphylaxis

The management of anaphylaxis depends primarily on the three "A's": Awareness, Avoidance and Action (i.e., epinephrine injection). Once the allergen has been pinpointed, avoidance is the key – especially being alert to hidden or accidental exposures. People must be fully informed about the severity of their allergy and have it evaluated by a reliable allergist, and must learn the correct emergency measures. While the best course for preventing anaphylaxis is obviously to avoid triggers – such as lobster, wasps or penicillin – the next best is to prepare ahead for a possible attack with a pocket self-injection kit – such as Ana-Kit, EpiPen or Ana-Guard – available by prescription. One injection may be enough, but a second dose, and even subsequent doses, may be needed 10 to 20 minutes later. (See below.)

People known to be at risk should also wear a medical-alert bracelet or necklet clearly stating "risk of anaphylaxis," the substance(s) to which they are allergic and the fact that they carry an injection kit. In addition, they should be sure the people around them – friends, relatives, co-workers – know what to do if they find someone in anaphylactic shock.

Taking preventive antihistamines (especially long-acting forms) before entering a situation with an exposure risk – going to a party, eating at a restaurant – may occasionally lessen the severity of an attack. But this practice is controversial; many experts believe that premedication masks the early warning signs of anaphylaxis (such as the hives and swelling or flushing), and may let the condition become very severe before the danger is recognized. "It cannot be emphasized enough," states one expert, "that epinephrine is the only proper treatment for anaphylaxis. Antihistamines take from half an hour to two hours to work and cannot save a life. Antihistamines are *not* a substitute for epinephrine; they are not strong enough to treat anaphylaxis, although they can be helpful in controlling the symptoms."

EpiPen and Use

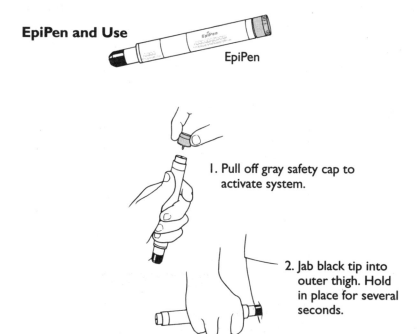

EpiPen

1. Pull off gray safety cap to activate system.

2. Jab black tip into outer thigh. Hold in place for several seconds.

Emergency Kits Save Lives

Some self-injector kits, such as the EpiPen, automatically inject a life-saving dose of epinephrine when the tip is pushed hard on the skin of the outside upper thigh. These are very easy to use. (An EpiPen Junior is available for children under 33 pounds – 15 kilos – in weight.) Other kits, such as the Ana-Kit, contain a preloaded syringe and needle that must be injected in the usual manner. A special plunger ensures that only one dose is injected at a time.

Kits should be kept out of direct sunlight, which may affect the drug, and very hot or cold conditions. Expired kits should be replaced.

All too often, people who have been prescribed self-injector kits don't have a kit on them when it's needed. They may be caught off guard – perhaps stung by a wasp at the pool, or unknowingly eating a bit of shrimp or peanut at a party – putting their lives in jeopardy. That's why, if you need a kit, you should *always* have it with you. Remember, though, that *emergency injection is no substitute for medical help.* It just "buys you time" until you can reach a physician or hospital.

Ana-kit

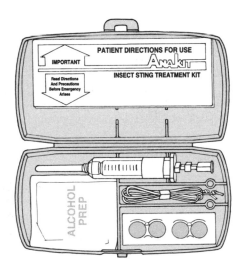

Act at the first hint of danger

Since there is not always much warning of an anaphylactic reaction, epinephrine should be self-injected at the *first hint* of a reaction, or on exposure to a known or suspected allergen. For someone who has collapsed in allergic shock on a previous occasion, the physician may suggest that an injection be administered immediately after a sting by a suspect insect, or contact with a dangerous drug or food, even before any reaction appears. "Whatever the reason for anaphylaxis," as one expert puts it, "it's better to act fast than to wait and be sure there will be a reaction. If you wait, it may be too late."

Exercise Can Provoke Anaphylaxis

Strenuous exercise occasionally produces a type of exercise-induced anaphylaxis, sometimes in combination with certain foods. Recognized since the 1970s, the problem is most often triggered by arduous exertion in joggers, runners, cyclists, soccer players, skiers and those engaging in vigorous aerobics. Its symptoms mimic anaphylaxis triggered by allergens – skin itching, diffuse flushing, often large (dime-sized) hives, swelling of the throat, hands and face, nausea and vomiting and lightheadedness. Attacks typically last 30 minutes to 4 hours. Choking and shock, even unconsciousness, can occur quickly – an emergency situation requiring immediate epinephrine injection. After an exercise-provoked episode, many people have a severe, persistent headache for 72 hours or longer.

In contrast to classic anaphylaxis, the exercise-induced form is not IgE-related but is due to direct stimulation of mast cells, which makes them release the mediators responsible for symptoms. Sometimes the itching, hives, swelling and other effects are triggered not only by exercise-generated heat and sweating but by *any* kind of heat – for instance, taking a sauna or hot shower. Known as *cholinergic urticaria,* these forms usually cause smaller hives and less dramatic symptoms, and are sometimes exacerbated by stress.

Food-dependent exercise attacks are another variant; they occur only if strenuous exercise is done within two to four hours of eating a meal, or after consuming specific foods (such as celery, wheat or shellfish), or when taking a particular medication such as ASA. The food or drug sets the scene and exercise finishes the job. One 25-year-old woman had episodes only on Friday evenings on the dance floor, after her escort had treated her to dinner. Her problem was resolved when she began eating dinner *after* dancing.

Some experts believe exercise-provoked anaphylaxis is becoming more common with the rising popularity of jogging, aerobics and other fitness programs. The people most susceptible are the allergy-prone. Attacks are more common or worse when exercise is done in humid conditions, in very cold air, during the pollen season or, in women, during a menstrual period.

First-aid guidelines for anaphylaxis

The Canadian Society for Allergy and Clinical Immunology, together with provincial affiliates and allergy organizations, has drafted a consensus statement to help simplify the management of anaphylaxis by the public, and especially by school staff.

The guidelines include the following measures:

- *Inject epinephrine* if available from an emergency kit. Rub the site vigorously afterwards to increase absorption.
- *Those known to be severely allergic* may be carrying an emergency kit such as the Ana-Kit or EpiPen, containing a preloaded syringe. In case of an allergic reaction, people can self-inject or be helped to do so.
- *Call emergency medical services immediately.*
- *Place a conscious person lying down* and elevate the feet by about twelve inches (30 cm), if possible.
- *Place an unconscious person* on his/her side to aid breathing.
- *Monitor the person and evaluate the need for CPR*, if you are trained in that procedure.

Diagnosing the condition may mean taking a "challenge test" – exercising on a treadmill or applying heat to see if symptoms appear. Blood tests sometimes show clearly elevated histamine levels during and after attacks.

Treatment of exercise-induced anaphylaxis is the same as for other anaphylactic reactions – injection of epinephrine, oxygen administration if needed, corticosteroids, antihistamines to blunt the severity and careful medical monitoring. Antihistamines have been used before exercise in attempts to forestall an allergic attack, but their use is *not* promoted as they cannot be relied on to stop the anaphylaxis.

Far more important are avoidance tactics – not exercising in humid conditions, avoiding vigorous activity for four hours after eating, heeding early warning signs and stopping exercise at the slightest hint of an oncoming attack – as soon as there's any skin itching, hives, flushing, swelling or dizziness. People prone to exercise-induced anaphylaxis should carry a self-injector kit, and always exercise with a companion who's aware of the problem and can help in an emergency. Sometimes, the reaction can be muted by starting an exercise program very slowly and working up to full speed.

FOUR

Diagnosing Allergies and Tracking Triggers

People commonly blame allergies for a whole range of imprecise symptoms, from fatigue, weakness and headache to depression and anxiety or behavior problems such as hyperactivity. The popular saying "I'm allergic to this or that" – to the furniture, broccoli or a certain plant – is a generic statement made without knowing or stopping to consider what an allergy really is. The goal in diagnosing allergies is to determine whether the reaction described is due to an allergic (immunological) response or to something else, and to try to pinpoint the specific allergen(s) that bring on the discomfort.

One problem in diagnosing an allergy is the common confusion between *allergy* and *toxicity*. Whereas toxins (poisons) – for example, cyanide or rattlesnake venom – harm almost everyone, allergens affect only about 15 to 20 percent of the North American population, but for this minority something as everyday as peanuts or cod can be deadly even in trace amounts.

Further confusion arises from the term "sensitivity." Some people are "sensitive" to (or dislike) the smell of garlic or a certain fragrance. That is *not* an allergic sensitivity. In allergic terms, "sensitivity" means that the immune system has been sensitized to a particular allergen and will react to it with a specific set of immunological changes. Although allergies can signal their presence in various ways and affect different parts of the body, an allergic reaction produces definite, reproducible and identifiable changes that can be evaluated – not vague, ill-defined complaints. Irritability, fatigue, anxiety, muscle aches, bedwetting and a host of other health problems frequently attributed to allergy are *not* immunological reactions – and *not* allergies.

Different Allergies Affect Different Body Sites
An allergic reaction can affect many parts of the body:
- *the nose and upper airways* – causing a runny nose, stuffiness and sneezing;
- *the lower bronchial passages (airways) and lungs* – producing chest tightness, wheezing, breathlessness and (in asthma) a cough;
- *the mouth and lips* – which may tingle, itch, burn or swell;
- *the throat* – which may become inflamed and constricted, jeopardizing breathing;
- *the eyes* – which may become red, puffy, watery and itchy;
- *the gastrointestinal tract* – producing nausea, vomiting and diarrhea;
- *the skin* – which can develop a rash, hives or dry, scaling sores (as in eczema) and flushing;
- *the entire body* – with multiple systems affected, producing airway obstruction and a precipitous drop in blood pressure (depriving the heart and brain of oxygen) leading to allergic shock and anaphylaxis.

Where Allergies May Strike

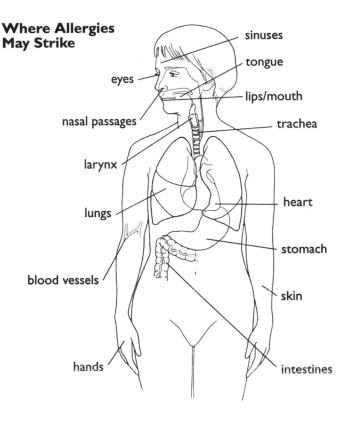

sinuses
tongue
eyes
lips/mouth
nasal passages
trachea
larynx
lungs
heart
stomach
blood vessels
skin
hands
intestines

Classic Signs and Symptoms of Allergy
Distressing but not life-endangering

- hives or a red, itchy rash
- sneezing, stuffy nose, clear nasal discharge
- tingling
- puffy face
- red, watery eyes
- gut spasms, maybe nausea and vomiting
- burning, itchy mouth/lips

Severe, possibly heralding anaphylaxis

- widespread hives
- face flushing

- swelling of tongue, larynx (voice box)
- altered voice, difficulty speaking
- constricted throat, trouble swallowing
- labored breathing, wheezing
- sense of doom
- irregular heartbeat
- drop in blood pressure
- loss of consciousness

Distinguishing Allergies from Non-allergic Reactions

If someone suspects an allergy, the first step is usually a visit to the family physician to find out whether the symptoms arise from an immune-system reaction or are due to some other disorder. Since some symptoms of allergy mimic those of other conditions, it's crucial to rule out other possibilities before diagnosing an allergy. Many intolerances and reactions to certain foods, drugs and other substances resemble but are *not* immunologically mediated reactions. Adverse responses blamed on allergies often arise from *non-immunological* causes – perhaps a specific disease or even pregnancy, which is known to cause hives, flushing and sneezing on occasion.

Physicians find that, in about half the cases investigated, the wheezing, runny eyes and nasal stuffiness don't stem from an allergy but from some other disorder, such as sinusitis or an eye infection. Rhinitis (a perpetually stuffy nose) is due to an allergy in only about 70 percent of cases examined. Only about 10 to 20 percent of reactions attributed to specific foods are real allergies; the rest are food intolerances.

In a few instances, it may not be necessary to discover whether symptoms arise from an allergic or a non-allergic disorder to plan treatment. For example, a troublesome reaction to ASA (aspirin) requires the same strategy – avoidance

– whatever the underlying mechanism. But distinguishing an allergic from a non-allergic reaction is usually essential for appropriate treatment. For example, to remedy a milk intolerance due to lack of the enzyme *lactase*, the person can consume milk products to which the missing enzyme has been added to make them digestible. But if the adverse symptoms stem from an allergy to cow's milk protein, cow's milk must be altogether avoided and replaced by a nutritionally sound substitute.

Taking a Medical and Family History

The medical and family history is the key to confirming an allergy and discovering its roots. The family physician, allergist, dermatologist or other specialist will take a thorough history, to obtain details about the circumstances of onset, duration and type of symptoms, family background, diet and

---

Allergy or not? Some telltale clues

- A clear discharge from a runny nose suggests allergy; a thick, colored discharge is more likely due to a viral or bacterial infection.
- Nasal itching and stuffiness around animals often indicate an allergy.
- Endless sneezing, nasal stuffiness and an itchy nose or red eyes at certain times of year suggest a seasonal pollen or mold allergy.
- Mild, intermittent wheezing suggests allergy, particularly in preschoolers. Chronic asthma is allergy-linked in 50 percent of children over age six.
- Eczema that's mild and patchy is probably not of allergic origin.
- Hives or swelling starting immediately after drinking milk or eating foods containing a common ingredient suggest a food allergy. Hives or swelling after eating a restaurant meal may stem from sensitivity to a flavor enhancer such as monosodium glutamate (MSG) or sulfite preservatives.
- If discomfort begins after certain medications are taken – such as antibiotics (especially penicillin, cephalosporins or sulfa drugs), arthritis medications or ASA (aspirin) – the problem may be a drug allergy.

lifestyle. Do other family members have any similar symptoms? Do the parents have an identified allergy or asthma? Allergic disorders often run in families, and having a relative with an allergy increases the chances that the sufferer's symptoms are also allergy-linked. The physician takes careful note of the allergy sufferer's home, school and work environment. By the end of the history-taking session, the physician should have a good picture of the reactions experienced by the sufferer and whether other family members have similar problems. Much valuable information can be obtained from a careful medical history; in many cases, it's all that's needed for diagnosis and for creating an effective allergy-management plan.

Tracing the Possible Triggers

Sometimes it's easy to deduce that someone has an allergy, and to work out what's causing it, just from a description of the symptoms. A woman who develops red, itchy eyes and begins to sneeze whenever she visits any friends with cats has almost certainly got a cat allergy. A man whose tongue starts to tingle and whose lips swell up whenever he eats eggs has likely got an egg allergy. In such clear-cut cases, although confirmation of the allergy is still needed, solving the problem is often largely a matter of common sense – avoiding the allergy-provoking substance and taking appropriate anti-allergy medications.

However, pinpointing an allergy isn't always so easy. Identifying what sets off an allergic reaction can be a long detective trail, especially if the allergens are unusual, if the reaction is a "delayed" type IV response, appearing hours or even days after exposure, or if a person suddenly reacts to a family pet or plant that has been around for a long time. The physician will search for clues to possible triggering substances and may test to see whether the suspected substances produce an observable skin reaction. Some people are convinced they are allergic to a certain food (such as shrimp or strawberries) but show no response on testing. In other cases, the person may have clear allergic symptoms but no idea what's causing them.

In tracking the offending substances, a wide variety of possible triggers may be investigated. As a cause of hay fever, suspected outdoor airborne triggers include pollens from trees, weeds and grasses, and spores from molds (fungi). Pollens, the male reproductive cells of various plants, are carried in the wind from spring to fall, and timing the onset and duration of allergic discomfort may reveal what specific pollens are to blame. Spores (reproductive cells) from fungi can cause problems from early spring right through to November or December. Pollens and molds wafted in from outside can also act as indoor triggers. (In the pollen season, one gram of indoor dust may contain as many as five to six million pollen grains.) Other indoor allergens to consider are dust mites, animal dander and cockroach (or other insect) parts.

Food allergens are sometimes hard to pin down, because the triggering substance may be a very minor ingredient in the food. Even vaccines (such as measles, influenza, mumps and yellow-fever vaccines) that contain traces of the egg in which they're grown can produce an allergic reaction in egg-sensitive persons.

Many medications – whether topical creams and ointments, oral or injected – cause allergies. In fact, drugs are among the most serious of allergy-causers. Substances that sensitize the skin and cause contact dermatitis include a huge list of plants, metals and chemicals, many of them in manufactured products. At last count the list of potentially sensitizing chemicals numbered 2,800, although only about 100 of them are common allergens.

Allergy triggers

Airborne:
Pollens
- grasses (e.g., timothy, rye, orchard and Kentucky)
- trees (e.g., ash, birch, elm, oak, hickory, pine, willow and mulberry)
- weeds (e.g., ragweed)

Molds
- fungal spores

Animal dander and secretions
- from cats, dogs, rabbits, rats, hamsters, mice, horses
- from birds (e.g., budgerigars, pigeons, chickens)

House dust mites: tiny, spider-like creatures that feed off shed skin cells and thrive in mattresses, upholstered furniture and carpets

Insect parts (e.g., from cockroaches, flies, midges, fleas)

Ingredients in commercial products (e.g., detergents, latex rubber, formaldehyde)

Cosmetic fragrances

Ingested:
Foods (most commonly cow's milk, eggs, nuts, peanuts, seafood)
Drugs (e.g., penicillin and other antibiotics – such as sulfonamides, cephalosporins, anesthetics, anti-inflammatories such as ASA, NSAIDs)

Injected:
Insect venom (e.g., wasps, hornets, bees, yellow jackets)
Injected medications, vaccines, hormones, contrast media (used in X-rays)

Skin-contact:
Cosmetics (e.g., ingredients in face creams, eye make-up, nail products)
Fragrances (e.g., in perfumes, skincare products)
Metals (e.g., nickel, chromium)
Plant components (e.g., urushiol in poison ivy, poison sumac; latex from rubber plants)
Chemicals (e.g., in dyes, resins, countless modern products)

Questions You May Be Asked

The examining physician will ask for a full description of the symptoms and when they first appeared. At what location and which time of year? What time of day do symptoms seem to be worst? Do they have a seasonal or daily pattern? Do you have a stuffy nose and sneeze a lot in certain seasons? Is there only one set of symptoms or are there different types? Do they come on soon after consuming a specific food or drink? Immediately, or after a day or two? Are symptoms worse at work or at home, or on weekends? Do the symptoms disappear when you're on holiday? Do they worsen in wet or dry weather? Questions about your environment at work and home give clues to the provocative allergens. Are there pets at home? Do you have friends or relatives with pets? Is your home new or old? Clean or dusty? The allergist may ask what *you* think causes the symptoms. If it proves particularly difficult to track elusive allergens, keeping a diary with details about where, how and when the symptoms appear may help pinpoint the cause.

Physical Diagnosis and Examination

A thorough physical checkup will help rule out diseases that might be causing the supposed allergy symptoms. The physician may examine your eyes, ears, nose, lungs and skin, perhaps also doing a breathing test and checking your nasal passages for evidence of inflammation. Skin and blood tests may also be done.

For example, when Craig was 35 years old he developed an itchy rash on his face and body. Thinking it might be an allergy, he stopped using the soap he had just bought, and tried eliminating other creams and face products. But nothing seemed to clear the rash. Finally he consulted a dermatologist, who thought it might be eczema – although, since Craig had no history of allergy, and eczema usually first appears in childhood, the diagnosis was doubtful. When the rash failed to clear with corticosteroid ointment, the dermatologist became suspicious and took a skin biopsy. The laboratory returned a diagnosis of *mycosis fungoides*, a rare form of cancer that has skin symptoms similar to eczema in its early stages. Fortunately, the disease was caught early enough for successful treatment and Craig's skin is now clear.

Allergy Tests

Skin tests, using extracts or ground-up bits of the suspected allergens, can help determine whether or not the problem is an allergy, and what triggers it. A bit of each test solution is put under the skin to see if it causes a reaction – a "weal and flare" (redness and swelling).

The first tests usually tried are prick or scratch tests, done in a row on the skin of the arm or back. A little of each suspected allergen is dabbed on the alcohol-cleaned skin, which is then pricked with a lancet (needle) through the allergy solution to get some solution under the skin. (The prick isn't deep enough to draw blood, but just lifts the skin surface.) After a while (usually a few minutes), if someone is sensitive to a specific allergen, the place where it was applied will become red and form a tiny hive. The development of this hivelike eruption is a "positive" test, indicating an allergy to that specific substance. Histamine solution is used as a "positive" control at one prick site – to produce a true allergic response – and saline solution at another spot as a negative control (no allergen present), to distinguish mere skin irritation from an allergic reaction.

Allergy skin tests are cheap and easy to do, and allow a broad range of allergens to be screened. However, allergists caution that the results of skin tests must be interpreted *together with* the patient's experiences and medical history. As mentioned earlier, skin tests should only be done by experienced allergists in locations with full emergency equipment, in case of unexpected or possibly severe reactions.

Other diagnostic methods are occasionally useful. The RAST (radioallergosorbent test) or the ELISA (enzyme-linked immunosorbent assay) may be used to measure the total amount of specific IgE antibodies in serum or blood. Sometimes, a combination of skin testing and serum IgE levels helps diagnose the condition. Another test, a provocation or "challenge" test, introduces a small amount of suspected allergen right into the nasal, bronchial or digestive passages. This poses a risk and should *only* be done in medical settings with full emergency capability and equipment nearby.

A Run-down on Skin Tests

- *The skin prick or puncture test* – the cheapest, safest, simplest and most commonly performed test for an allergy – is done in an emergency-equipped doctor's office, takes only a few minutes and can identify an IgE antibody reaction, giving a good index of allergic response. A few drops of specially prepared common allergen extracts are introduced beneath the skin on the forearm or back, and the skin sites are examined after 15 minutes to see if there's any "weal and flare," indicating sensitivity to any of the allergens.

  Although skin prick tests can't prove that a certain agent is causing the allergy, and don't test for non-IgE allergies, they do test for sensitization and detect the presence of specific IgE antibodies. For example, one girl with severe hay fever developed a red spot where pollen extracts from timothy, june and orchard grasses were applied, but not where other pollens were applied. Skin prick tests should *not* be done soon after taking an antihistamine, which can suppress the response, or for widespread eczema or chronic hives. All allergy tests should be done by experienced testers who can interpret the results properly and have appropriate emergency help nearby.

- *Scratch tests* are similar to skin prick tests, except that the skin is first scratched and then a drop of the suspected allergen extract is applied. These are no more sensitive or specific than the gentler skin prick tests, and can leave scars, so they are less often done.

- *The intradermal test* injects a tiny amount of allergen into the skin. Although more sensitive, it's less specific, difficult to do on children and more likely to produce adverse reactions.

- *Patch tests* examine substances for their ability to cause contact dermatitis. They are most often done for skin rashes that might stem from various chemicals, cosmetics, creams or ointments. The allergen extracts are put on the skin (usually on the upper back) and the test sites are covered with patches and later observed for red spots or hives. The patches are removed two to three days later and the sites are inspected for redness and inflammation, denoting sensitivity. A standard battery of patch tests might include nickel, chromium, rubber, certain plant extracts, drugs, cosmetic ingredients and other chemicals.

Note that skin testing may not be appropriate for people who have had life-threatening allergic reactions, or who have skin rashes on large areas of their bodies. In these cases, blood tests may be more safely used instead.

Blood Tests
Blood tests are more expensive than skin tests but not more

sensitive, so they are only used when skin testing could be dangerous or is impractical for other reasons.

The radioallergosorbent test (RAST) measures allergen-specific IgE levels. A positive result shows that the person is sensitized to the particular allergen but does not prove that that allergen is the cause of the symptoms. The RAST is roughly equivalent to the skin prick test: a sample of blood is added to the suspected allergen and IgE activity is identified by radiolabeled (radioactive) anti-IgE antibodies. Because the RAST is carried out on a blood sample in the laboratory, it avoids the risk of severe reactions and causes less patient anxiety. It's used mainly when skin tests cannot easily be done – for instance, if the person to be tested:

- is taking antihistamines (which can mask the weal-and-flare response);
- has severe eczema;
- has *dermatographism*, a condition in which the skin reacts to anything and everything;
- is very afraid of prick tests.

Total serum IgE tests measure the total amount of IgE in a blood sample. This method is hardly ever used because it does not reveal *which* substances cause the allergy, or its severity, and people with normal IgE readings may still be allergic. Blood IgE measurements alone cannot diagnose an allergy, but elevated blood IgE may suggest one. For example, a high blood IgE level in a child with eczema may help pinpoint the eczema as allergy-related.

Food Challenge and Dietary Tests

The double-blind challenge test is the only scientifically validated test to see if a certain food or drug is causing allergic problems. The food ingredient to be tested may be freeze-dried and hidden in a gelatin capsule that the patient swallows whole; physician and patient wait to see whether symptoms appear when the gelatin dissolves in the stomach, releasing the test ingredient. As a control the person instead swallows a gelatin capsule containing a placebo (with no allergen). If, after a number of challenges, symptoms have appeared only with the real food and not with the placebo capsule, it is likely that the suspected food is an allergy-provoker.

It's essential to this test that neither the allergist nor the person tested know whether the suspected food or the placebo is being swallowed. Allergy-like symptoms can arise from the "placebo effect," when the patient is convinced that a certain food causes problems such as nausea and therefore develops those problems. If the allergist knows which food capsule is real, the patient may subconsciously pick up clues to that information and react accordingly.

Food challenge tests are time-consuming and are usually done only for research purposes or when there is doubt that a food is causing symptoms.

Open dietary challenges are more likely to be tried than double-blind food challenges, to diagnose a food allergy or determine whether someone has outgrown one. For an open challenge, the physician places a tiny flake of the suspected food on the person's lips and waits 20 minutes to see what happens. If no symptoms such as tingling or itching occur, then a little more food is tried, then a little more. If the person can eat a normal amount without a reaction, it's assumed that the allergy doesn't exist or has been outgrown.

Elimination diets, often used to test for food allergies in the past, are now seldom used. The person was placed on a diet consisting of just a few foods – ones that rarely cause allergies, such as lamb, turkey, tuna, squash, rice, sweet potato, peaches and pears – until all symptoms disappeared. Then one new food at a time was reinstated, and the person was carefully observed. This procedure is very tedious, requiring meticulous compliance.

One frequent problem with elimination diets is that they don't allow for the placebo effect. Take Margie, who read a magazine article claiming that chocolate caused headaches. She had been having frequent headaches in the last few months, and eating a lot of chocolate, one of her favorite sweets. To stop the headaches she was willing to give up every type of chocolate. Sure enough, her symptoms disappeared and she felt much better. However, whenever she slipped up and ate chocolate her symptoms would return; she would feel irritable and snippy, and have headaches. Several months later, her headaches returned even though she wasn't eating chocolate. Margie and her husband decided to test the chocolate hypothesis. They went to an allergist who performed a double-blind challenge test, alternating real chocolate in capsules with dummy chocolate. After swallowing the chocolate capsule, Margie often felt irritable and headachy. However, these symptoms also occurred after she consumed the dummy candy. On other occasions she would eat the chocolate and have no symptoms or she would eat the placebo and have symptoms. The physician performed the challenges several times, until Margie could see clearly that her symptoms had no logical relationship to her diet. Whatever was causing her headaches, it wasn't chocolate.

Difficulties in Interpreting Allergy Tests
Although prick and patch tests add information to the medical history, such tests used alone can be very misleading. They are no substitute for painstaking, detailed history-taking that tries to correlate the symptoms with the person's experience and exposure to potential allergens. For example, a large

number of people with no allergic symptoms whatsoever test positive to allergens put into the skin. "False positive" reactions can have unfortunate consequences. A skin test that wrongly pinpoints eggs as a cause of eczema, for example, might needlessly persuade someone to give up eggs. Worse still, skin tests can be positive to a whole range of foods, only one of which is actually causing allergic symptoms. Parents whose child tests positive to eggs, milk, wheat and nuts may limit the child's diet, cutting out or reducing the intake of several essential nutrients.

On the other hand, dietary allergy tests can narrow the field from a vast range of possibly allergenic foods to a limited number, and then a challenge test or an elimination diet can further narrow the field to the most likely offender. For example, in the above case, where the child's skin showed a strong positive reaction to eggs, milk, wheat and nuts, challenge tests and elimination diets might indicate which trigger caused the symptoms.

Pete, an allergy sufferer who is now 28, agrees that allergy tests should be used judiciously. When he was 12 years old, his parents took him to an allergist who tested him with a huge battery of allergens. As Pete recalls, "the skin test was horrible – both my forearms from wrist to elbow were covered with huge welts and itchy swellings. According to the skin tests I was allergic to everything – several kinds of tree pollen and some insects, every kind of furry or feathery animal. But I didn't really see the point of all this knowledge, like knowing I was allergic to horses. So what? The only time I ever saw a horse, it was going down a street with a cop on its back."

Allergy Tests Best Avoided

Nontraditional allergy practitioners and clinical ecologists frequently offer unconventional allergy tests, often in conjunction with therapies based on the test results. Some tests of no proven value include:

- *the cytotoxic test,* in which drops of blood put on a microscope slide are mixed with dried food extracts. The white blood cells are scrutinized for changes alleged to indicate a particular allergy. Blood cells disintegrate or become less mobile in positive reactions, according to practitioners;
- *provocation-neutralization testing and therapy,* in which the person is given an increasing dose of allergen by injection or by mouth until symptoms supposedly appear (by provocation), and then the dose is decreased until symptoms disappear (by neutralization) – of dubious value;
- *the pulse test,* in which the pulse rate is measured following exposure to supposed allergens. Advocates of these tests claim the pulse rate increases by 20 percent following ingestion of allergy-causing foods;
- *applied kinesiology,* in which a vial of allergen is placed on the skin and muscle strength is measured to indicate the strength of the body's response.

Generally considered unscientific, these tests are opposed by most medical allergists because there is no established body of research on which they are based, or which convincingly explains how the tests work. It has not been shown, for example, that allergies increase or decrease muscle strength, or that an allergic reaction makes blood cells behave in an observably unusual way. On the contrary, studies find that provocation-neutralization and cytotoxic testing cannot distinguish between symptoms caused by a supposed allergen and those due to a placebo. Moreover, these methods can do harm to the person's quality of life and lead to malnutrition, or mask the diagnosis of other disorders.

FIVE

Managing Allergies

W ith one in five North Americans suffering from some kind of allergy, managing the disorder is big business. Air-cleaning filters and other aids are flooding the market to help reduce allergic distress. Also, better understanding of the allergic mechanism has given us many medications to relieve or block the allergic process.

The best way to start managing allergies is to follow a few simple rules, and to make sure any help and advice come from reliable, well-qualified medical experts. First and foremost, once an allergy has been correctly diagnosed and the suspected allergen pinpointed, the key strategy is "environmental control" – trying to avoid or reduce exposure to the provocative agents. When it's not possible to completely avoid an allergen, a roster of medications is available to help relieve symptoms. Immunotherapy (allergy injections) can prevent attacks or curb the allergic reaction in some cases.

Getting Expert Advice

In many cases, people manage their allergy simply by taking over-the-counter preparations as needed, perhaps with the advice of the family physician or pharmacist. More severe cases may require referral to a specialist such as a dermatologist, respirologist, immunologist or allergist. Getting advice from a licensed allergist – a physician with specialized postgraduate training in immunology and allergy management – rather than just trying to "tough it out" is the best idea (see the resource section at the end of this book). For those prone to anaphylaxis, obtaining expert medical advice is a must – preferably from physicians certified in clinical immunology and allergy.

People who consult an allergist should check whether the specialist is a medical doctor with the required postgraduate training. Non-accredited or self-nominated "allergists" may offer therapies that have little or no scientific merit and could be harmful. For example, in Britain so-called allergy testing is springing up in grocery stores, where people can have their allergy "diagnosed" by a skin test that's of dubious value unless medically interpreted in the context of the history and observed symptoms. Allergy sufferers are advised to check that any allergist consulted belongs to an accredited organization such as the American Academy of Allergy, Asthma and Immunology or the Canadian Society of Allergy and Clinical Immunology, and is recognized as a certified clinical immunologist by this organization.

A Three-Pronged Attack on Allergies

The key methods of treating and managing allergies are avoidance, pharmacotherapy (with appropriate medications) and immunotherapy (allergy injections).

Avoidance, or "environmental control" – strategy number one – means avoiding allergens known to trigger the allergic symptoms. It may involve avoiding specific foods, pollens, molds, animals or allergy-provoking medications, and may even demand changing jobs to avoid an allergy-causing substance such as a latex or hair dye.

Pharmacotherapy, the second line of allergy treatment, can now rely on a wide variety of medications. Antihistamines – which block histamine receptors and dampen or stop the effects of histamine – are the mainstay of today's treatment.

Decongestants and corticosteroid nasal sprays are also crucial weapons in the allergy-relieving drug arsenal. For asthma, corticosteroid inhalers are now widely prescribed as first-line drugs. Other asthma medications include bronchodilators (airway wideners) for occasional symptom relief, and non-steroidal anti-inflammatory drugs. Still other medications act on other aspects of the immune reaction – for example, cromolyn suppresses mast cell "degranulation" and helps to stop symptoms from surfacing.

Immunotherapy, or "desensitizing" allergy shots – the third weapon in treating allergies – is suitable for selected people with certain allergies. It's the one form of therapy that alters immune-system activity and offers the chance of a cure for IgE-dependent allergies. It involves a lengthy course (up to five years) of regular injections. Immunotherapy is used primarily for cases where avoidance and medication fail to control symptoms, and is especially helpful for those allergic to insect venom, dust mites and specific pollens, and for a very few people with asthma.

The ultimate goal of allergy treatment is to find some way to control the components of the immune system that orchestrate the allergic reaction. "Basically," notes one Baltimore allergist, "we would like to inhibit or turn off the activity of the 'bad' cells, which stimulate mast cells and provoke the inflammatory response." Although a cure isn't yet possible, well-tailored therapy can control most allergy symptoms, except for very severe or unusual ones, so that allergy sufferers can generally live in reasonable comfort with their affliction.

Making Avoidance Work

Avoidance of allergens may mean not eating eggs or seafood, giving away a much-loved pet, exercising only at certain times of day (when pollen counts are low), altering home decor and furnishings or trying to change school and work environments. For those with allergic rhinitis – whether seasonal (like hay fever) or year-round (like a dust-mite or cat allergy) – allergen avoidance may entail stringent efforts to make the home low in allergens, by reducing the level of common triggers such as pollens, molds, dust mites, cockroach parts and animal dander. The number of control measures needed to keep symptoms at bay depends on the type of allergy and the severity of symptoms. (See Chapters Six and Seven for details on making homes more allergen-free.)

Allergen Avoidance May Involve:
For those with seasonal rhinitis (hay fever):
- trying to keep allergy-triggering pollens out of the house by closing windows and installing air-conditioners;
- making the house as pollen-free as possible;

Clues that the indoor environment may be at fault

- a perpetually stuffy, sneezing, itchy nose
- sore, red or puffy eyes when you're at home (possibly improved when you're away from home – although dust mites can be anywhere!)
- more than one member of the household suffering similar symptoms
- reduction in symptoms when you're away from home for a few days, or on vacation
- distress that's worse in certain parts of the house, especially in the basement – a possible sign of a mold or cockroach allergy
- symptoms that are worse at certain times of the year – perhaps when you first turn on the furnace and dry out the air

- minimizing outdoor activity during a particular tree, grass, or weed pollen season, or restricting it to times of day when pollen counts are lowest;

For those with year-round (perennial) rhinitis:

- enclosing mattresses in zippered plastic covers or a vapor-permeable, allergen-proof fabric;
- damp-wiping mattress covers every two weeks;
- washing bedding often, in very hot water;
- eliminating molds by keeping bathrooms and basement as dry as possible, and damp-mopping with household cleaner or a bleach solution;
- placing objects that accumulate dust in drawers or closed cabinets;
- vacuuming carpets weekly or replacing them with wooden floors;

For those with a food allergy:

- avoiding all foods containing even traces of an offending allergen;

For those allergic to animal dander:

- getting rid of a pet;

For those allergic to cockroach parts:

- closing entry points into the home;
- using bait to kill roaches;
- keeping the kitchen clean;
- covering all food and promptly disposing of garbage;

For those with contact dermatitis or a product allergy:

- avoiding contact with any items that cause allergic skin problems (eczema, rash or hives).

Making Your Home Less Allergenic

If something in your home is triggering an allergy, altering the home environment may be an essential part of management.

What if your pet is your best friend?

In the U.S., two million people allergic to their pets apparently prefer to sneeze and sniffle through the year rather than part with a cat or dog. Allergists usually emphasize that people with a severe pet allergy that can't be controlled with medications and good house-cleaning should get rid of the animal. But for some people it's heart-wrenching to give up a pet. If the allergy is mild, symptoms may be suppressed by making sure the pet is banned from the bedroom, and by using medications such as antihistamines and corticosteroids.

Keeping the animal outdoors as much as possible may help, but this is debatable, and not always practical. Room air cleaners with HEPA (high-efficiency particulate air) filters can reduce airborne cat or dog allergens. Although allergic reactions are less common with dogs than with cats, the same advice holds – keep the dog outdoors as much as possible, wash it weekly and banish it from the allergic person's bedroom.

Claims that you have to strip the house completely are usually an exaggeration. Meticulous cleaning to make it as dust-free and mold-free as possible is enough. Those with rhinitis due to molds, dust mites or other indoor allergens may feel better if they simply keep the home cool, with low humidity (below 30 percent), and ensure good ventilation. As one Canadian allergist notes, "If we could only persuade people to run their houses cooler – below 20°C (68°F) – and drier, then dust-mite, cockroach and fungal problems would decrease. For someone with asthma, these changes can make all the difference. You don't have to spend a fortune to take sensible measures. No sense in undertaking major renovations if they're not likely to help." This expert recounts the example of someone whose family spent many thousands of dollars refurbishing their house – installing a new ventilation system, new insulation, new flooring and so on – to try to make it allergen-free. He calls this "overkill."

How Antihistamines Work

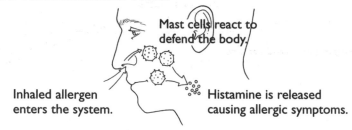

Mast cells react to defend the body.

Inhaled allergen enters the system.

Histamine is released causing allergic symptoms.

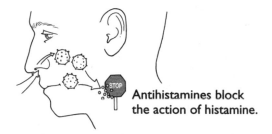

Antihistamines block the action of histamine.

Pharmacotherapy

These days, well-tailored, individualized pharmacotherapy with one or more allergy medications can relieve most symptoms, except for the most severe. There is an arsenal of drugs to choose from which, properly used, achieve good control for most allergy sufferers.

Antihistamines block the effects of histamine – one of the key mediators released by mast cells during an allergic attack. Antihistamines bind to receptors on the target organs, reducing allergic inflammation. A large variety of antihistamines is now available to choose from, in consultation with a physician. They are referred to as H_1 or H_2 blockers, depending on the kind of histamine receptor sites they bind to. Most of those used for allergies are H_1 blockers. The H_2 blockers – such as cimetidine (Tagamet), ranitidine (Zantac) and famotidine (Pepcid) – block mainly gastric symptoms.

Anti-inflammatories, particularly corticosteroids – usually from an inhaled spray or "puffer" – are very helpful in

Antihistamines

Generic name	Some brand names	Formulation and dose	Kind of blocker	Sedative effects/ drowsiness	Anticholinergic effects**
First-generation antihistamines					
Azatadine	Optimine	tablets twice daily	H_1	moderate	moderate
Brompheniramine	Dimetane, Dimetapp	syrup, tablets every 4 hours	H_1	low	moderate
Chlorpheniramine	Aller-Chlor*, Chlor-Trimeton, Allermine*, Chlor-Tripolon†, Chlorate†, Histex* Chlor-4*,	tablets, syrup every 4 hours; sprays	H_1	low	moderate
Clemastine	Tavist	tablets twice daily	H_1	moderate	high
Cyproheptadine	Periactin	tablets, syrup	H_1	low	moderate
Diphenhydramine	Allerdryl†, Benahist*, Allernixt†, Benylin Benadryl,	capsules, elixir every 6 hours	H_1	high	high
Hydroxyzine	Atarax	capsules, syrup	H_1	moderate	low
Pheniramine	Inhiston*, Triaminic†	tablets	H_1	moderate	moderate
Promethazine	Phenergan	tablets, liquid	H_1	high	high
Tripelennamine	Pyribenzamine	tablets	H_1	moderate	low to none
Second-generation antihistamines					
Astemizole	Hismanal	tablets/suspension once daily	H_1	low to none	low to none
Cetirizine	Cetirizine*, Reactine†	tablets once daily	H_1	low	low
Ketotifen	Zaditen†	tablets/syrup	H_1	low	low
Levocabastine	Livostin	spray	H_1	low	low
Loratadine	Claritin†	tablets/syrup	H_1	low to none	low to none
Terfenadine	Seldane	tablets/syrup	H_1	low to none	low to none

*Available in U.S. only.

†Available in Canada only.

**Anticholinergic effects are mouth dryness, blurred vision, urinary retention, constipation.

Note: Competing athletes who use over-the-counter allergy medications – especially those that act as stimulants (eg., ephedrine) – could be disqualified. Check the status of such drugs with an expert.

suppressing the inflammatory aspects of an allergic reaction, reducing the swelling and discomfort. They are widely used for allergic rhinitis and asthma.

Mast-cell stabilizers such as cromolyn and nedocromil are weak anti-inflammatory agents that partially prevent basophils and mast cells from releasing their potent mediators. They are helpful for preventing or treating mild to moderate asthma, eye symptoms and allergic rhinitis.

Bronchodilators are invaluable in relieving the symptoms of asthma, helping to relax smooth muscle and widen inflamed and narrowed airways. However, they are *not* recommended for regular use or without additional, anti-inflammatory inhalers, except in very mild cases. They should *not* be relied upon as number-one asthma antidotes as they can cover up symptoms of severe asthmatic lung inflammation, which needs a different approach and different medications. (See Chapter Nine.)

Antihistamines Old and New

Antihistamines block or mute various allergy symptoms, including hives, inflammation and the nasal and eye discomfort of hay fever. These medications come as so-called older or first-generation (more sedating) types and second-generation (less sedating) forms. The older ones have more annoying side-effects such as drowsiness, urinary retention, mouth dryness and vision blurring. The second-generation forms tend to cause less (or no) drowsiness or mouth drying, but some have contraindications that prohibit their use in certain cases. The choice is very individual; some people try many types before finding the most effective antihistamine with the fewest side-effects for them.

One common mistake is to take antihistamines only as "rescue" medications, when symptoms worsen. Antihistamines are most effective if started as soon as or *just before* symptoms start – in anticipation of allergy symptoms, or even before exposure – for example, at least half an hour before visiting a friend with a cat. Use should continue for long enough after exposure. Side-effects are less of a problem if the medication is taken at bedtime, when its sedative properties are a bonus.

First-generation antihistamines are still popular, and the sedative side-effects often disappear or lessen within the first week or so. However, first-generation antihistamines depress the brain and CNS (central nervous system), reducing alertness and reaction time as well as the ability to concentrate. They must be used with caution, as they diminish performance and driving skills, and can seriously impair coordination. They should be used with particular caution by the elderly, and should not be used by people with asthma, glaucoma, breathing problems, prostate trouble or certain other medical conditions, or by pregnant women, or by children under 12 without medical advice. Side-effects worsen in combination with alcohol, which is also a brain depressant, and the two together have been implicated in some traffic fatalities, due to the driver's drowsiness and slowed reaction time.

First-generation antihistamines also cause *anticholinergic* effects, producing a dry mouth, blurred vision, urine retention and sometimes impotence. Overdose of certain first-generation sedating antihistamines can produce serious CNS-depressant effects, with coma, seizures, hallucination and heart problems.

Second-generation antihistamines are generally longer-lasting and less sedating, with fewer anticholinergic effects, and one (cetirizine) also has anti-inflammatory benefits. Others (ketotifen, terfenadine, loratadine and azatadine) have some mast-cell stabilizing effects. Developed specifically to be non-sedating, they are "lipophobic" (water-repelling) and so unable to cross from the bloodstream into the brain itself, so they

Other Allergy Medications

Generic name	Some brand names	Formulation	Action
Corticosteroids			
Beclomethasone	Beclovent, Beconase	spray (mouth)	anti-inflammatory
Betamethasone	Betacort, Betatrex*, Betnovate	cream	anti-inflammatory
Budesonide	Rhinocort	spray	anti-inflammatory
Methylprednisolone	Depo-Medrol, Medrol	injection	anti-inflammatory
Flunisolide	AeroBid†, Nasalide, Bronalide, Rhinalar	spray, eyedrops	anti-inflammatory
Triamcinolone	Aristocort, Kenacort, Kenalog†	spray, cream	anti-inflammatory
Fluticasone	Flonase	spray	anti-inflammatory
Mast-cell stabilizers			
Cromolyn/cromoglycate	Intal, Opticrom, Nasalcrom†, Rynacrom†	spray, eyedrops	mast-cell blocker
Nedocromil	Tilade	spray	mast-cell blocker
Decongestants (some combined with other ingredients)			
Ephedrine/ pseudoephedrine	Sudafed	tablets, syrup	CNS stimulant
Naphazoline	Privine	spray, eyedrops	vasoconstrictor
Oxymetazoline	Dristan Long Lasting Nasal Mist†, Duration Nasal Spray*	spray	vasoconstrictor
Xylometazoline	Otrivin	spray, drops	vasoconstrictor
Phenylpropanolamine	Coricidin, Dimetapp, Sinutab	tablets, syrup, spray	CNS stimulant

CNS = central nervous system.   *Available in U.S. only.   †Available in Canada only.

have less sedative, performance-reducing and CNS effects. But some of them take longer to work than first-generation products – 1 to 3 hours for terfenadine (Seldane) and up to 2 days for astemizole (Hismanal). So some people who want instant relief may still prefer first-generation products, which start acting 15 to 30 minutes after ingestion. However, the latest second-generation products – loratadine (Claritin) and cetirizine (Reactine) – have a rapid onset of action, within 30 minutes. Cetirizine is somewhat sedating but has very few side-effects, and it's the drug of choice for elderly allergic people and those with liver ailments.

Some Newer Antihistamines Also Call for Caution

Some of the second-generation antihistamines, especially astemizole (Hismanal) and terfenadine (Seldane), have been associated with serious cardiovascular effects and heart-rhythm disturbances in a few cases, so it's essential not to exceed the recommended dose. Combined with some antibiotics such as erythromycin, terfenadine and astemizole can produce heartbeat irregularities. So anyone on these antibiotics should choose another antihistamine. Liver problems can also occur or be worsened in those taking either of these two antihistamines if they're also taking medications that inhibit the liver's metabolism of antihistamines – such as the antifungals ketoconazole, itraconazole and fluconazole (Diflucan), as well as certain antibiotics such as erythromycin or clarithromycin (Biaxin), the anti-ulcer drug cimetidine or disulfiram (Antabuse). People with heart, liver or kidney disorders, the elderly, those with cancer and people on antidepressants should not use second-generation antihistamines without medical advice. These antihistamines also haven't been shown to be safe for use during pregnancy or lactation. In general, second-generation antihistamines should be taken with a physician's advice, and package information should be read carefully. In the U.S., terfenadine and astemizole are prescription drugs, and the Food and Drug Administration is suggesting removal of terfenadine (Seldane) from the market. In Canada these two antihistamines are nonprescription products, but are only available on request from the pharmacist, who explains the precautions needed.

Pros and Cons of Immunotherapy

"Desensitization," "hyposensitization" and "immunotherapy" are interchangeable terms for the injection of allergen extracts to reduce the severity of allergic reactions. Allergen immunotherapy, which has been around since the turn of the century, is the only allergy treatment that actually alters immune-system activity. Although not a certain cure, immunotherapy can help to reduce symptoms in some types of allergy. Better-purified allergen extracts, and new U.S. and Canadian guidelines for their use, are improving the efficacy of immunotherapy – provided the right allergen extracts are used, in high enough doses. Although its mechanism is not yet fully understood, immunotherapy dampens the allergic reaction, possibly by suppressing IgE production.

Despite the high demand for allergy injections, the method is considered suitable for only a few specific allergies – those due to certain pollens, insect-sting venoms and possibly dust mites – and only in selected cases. For severe insect-venom allergies, it's often the treatment of choice. But immunotherapy is not yet suitable for food allergies, nor are allergy shots any use for eczema or hives – which may in fact be aggravated by them.

However, immunotherapy is subject to misuse and overuse, and some providers don't conform to the accepted guidelines. "Immunotherapy raises some emotional issues often based more on bias than on science," notes one member of the Canadian Society of Allergy and Clinical Immunology (CSACI). "Critics worry about the overuse of allergy injections. Charges that immunotherapy is overprescribed are beamed mainly at physicians who use it as first-line treatment, rather than reserving it for use after avoidance and medications fail to relieve allergic distress." A U.S. allergist points out that "immunotherapy is very effective when well done, but at our center it's considered suitable for only 10 percent of our allergic population, if that." The American Academy of Allergy, Asthma and Immunology estimates that, at most, one in ten people treated for allergies to inhaled substances qualifies for immunotherapy.

CSACI has recently established guidelines for immunotherapy, resembling those of American authorities. To qualify for desensitizing injections, someone must have an identified IgE-mediated reaction to a specific allergen with recognizable symptoms that have lasted at least two years, and insufficient relief obtained through allergen avoidance and medication.

"Allergy shots are not a substitute for removing the cat," comments one immunologist. "And people with ambiguous or unreliable skin tests should *not* be put on shots." Before starting immunotherapy, the physician should make every attempt to educate the allergy sufferer about the role of preventive measures and the proper use of prescribed medications. Studies show that in selected patients, both adults and children (at least five years old), immunotherapy can abolish or reduce symptoms of allergic rhinitis due to pollens (tree, grass and ragweed) and dust mites – even in those who don't respond to drug treatment. The guidelines do *not* endorse short-term immunotherapy before the allergy season, when allergic problems are anticipated. "In the case of allergic rhinitis," explains one allergist, "allergy injections are no longer necessary for most sufferers because there are safe, effective medications that work well. In those allergic to only one or two pollens, and provided pure, effective extracts are available, immunotherapy may help, but avoidance and drug treatment are usually enough."

If allergy injections are done correctly, the spinoff is not only allergy relief but also less inflammation, less damage to the lining tissues and fewer bouts of sinusitis and respiratory infections. To be successful, though, high doses of allergen extract must be given. A "shotgun" approach, with a mixture of many (often crude) extracts and low doses, doesn't work.

Critical to success is the purity of the allergen extracts. Whenever possible, standardized allergens should be used, and their potency assessed. At present, there are standard extracts only for dust-mite, cat-dander, bee-venom, ragweed, grass and birch allergens. Maintenance shots are usually continued every three to four weeks for five years, but no longer. Although the criteria for this cutoff are not well established, some studies show long-term remission after five years. If there's no symptom relief after two years, the injections should be discontinued.

Overall, there are few adverse effects of immunotherapy. But it is more time-consuming, inconvenient and uncomfortable than medication, and there are no good indicators to predict who will do well, or laboratory tests to show when injections should be discontinued. Anaphylaxis is the most serious risk, and deaths have occurred from errors – wrong allergen extract, wrong person, wrong dose. In one study of deaths from immunotherapy, the doctors' offices had no emergency equipment or epinephrine on hand. "Such tragedies are avoidable with proper training of healthcare professionals," says one emergency-medicine expert. "Alertness and vigilance are the key. Even the receptionist in a medical practice should notice if someone keeps clearing the throat after receiving the injection, or seems shaky and flushed – not wait for total collapse."

In the United Kingdom, because of deaths from immunotherapy, the procedure has been largely discontinued since 1986, when the Committee for the Safety of Medicines recommended it be used only for strictly defined conditions (such as allergy to bee stings) and done only in specialty centers with full emergency equipment available.

A Summary of Immunotherapy
Immunotherapy is advised only for:
- *severe, IgE-mediated allergic rhinitis* (if it's seasonal it must have lasted two or more years) in which allergen avoidance and proper medication have not managed to control the symptoms;
- *IgE-mediated anaphylactic reactions to insect stings,* using purified venom from yellow jackets, yellow hornets, white-faced hornets, wasps and honeybees, or whole-body extracts for fire-ant allergy. Allergy injections with insect venom are 95 percent protective against anaphylactic reactions to these insects;
- *some cases of IgE-mediated asthma,* when there is a clear link between exposure to the allergen and asthma symptoms, if symptoms have persisted for two or more allergy seasons despite avoidance and proper use of anti-inflammatories. But many allergists consider immunotherapy controversial and only *very rarely* useful for asthma.

Potential risks of immunotherapy
- swelling and soreness at the injection site
- anaphylaxis – the only serious risk
- sensitization to the allergen, if therapy is wrongly used

Allergy management in pregnancy

In pregnancy, rhinitis or nasal allergies can be aggravated by increased blood flow, blood-vessel dilation and increased mucus secretion – mainly in mid and late term. Hives rarely start up in pregnancy, because hormonal changes mute the allergic response. About one-third of asthma cases worsen, one-third improve and one-third remain unchanged. Medications passed as "safe" for use in pregnancy are considered free of harmful effects on the developing fetus. Some broncho-inhalers such as beclomethasone, cromolyn and inhaled steroids are considered safe for expectant mothers. Cromolyn is often the first medication considered for treating rhinitis in pregnancy.

Antihistamines are not necessarily safe to take while you are pregnant, but if you need them a physician can advise you on what's best. They should be avoided particularly during the third trimester, because of the risk of severe reactions (such as seizures) in premature infants and newborns. Astemizole and terfenadine should not be taken by pregnant women. Chlorpheniramine and diphenhydramine are considered relatively safe but not recommended without consultation with a specialist. Antihistamines are generally contraindicated for women who are breastfeeding because of the risk of harmful effects on the baby – mainly with the first-generation types, which pass into breastmilk and could cause respiratory depression, sleep apnea and "crib death" (sudden infant death syndrome), especially in newborns and premature infants.

Although immunotherapy should not be started in pregnancy, it's generally considered safe to continue if you become pregnant during the course of the shots. Anaphylaxis is rare in pregnancy, but if it occurs it's life-threatening to both mother and fetus. It should be treated the same way as for non-pregnant women, even though epinephrine may reduce the blood flow to the baby.

Allergy injections are not recommended for:

- food allergies (such treatment is considered dangerous);
- severe, uncontrolled asthma (also dangerous);
- children under age five;
- people with urticaria (hives) or atopic dermatitis (eczema), as these conditions may be aggravated rather than relieved;
- people whose medical history, physical exam and laboratory tests do not indicate an IgE-mediated allergy;

- those in whom previous, properly administered immunotherapy has failed;
- those who have already had a five-year course of allergy injections;
- those whose symptoms have not abated after two years of allergy injections;
- those on beta-blocker medications, which can create a *serious risk* of severe reactions;
- those with coexisting autoimmune disease such as rheumatoid arthritis, serum sickness or lupus erythematosus.

Note: The use of bacterial extracts, histamine shots or urine extracts is absolutely *contraindicated.*

The Future of Allergy Management

Given the limitations of current allergy treatment – the reluctance of some of those affected to take nonstop medication, the fact that some people don't use their medications as they should, the side-effects of some drugs – scientists are urgently researching new allergy therapies. Recent insights into the complexities of the allergic response – how the immune system's T-cells mastermind the allergic cascade – are opening new avenues to prevention.

Many of the methods being developed depend on "downregulating" or switching off the action of the cells that spark the allergic response. Understanding how the immune system works in allergies may pave the way to better therapy, cure or anti-allergy vaccines. Already special peptides (protein fragments) have been found that can turn off some aspects of the allergic process. Another route is to stop mast cells from releasing their mediators.

Possible ways to block or turn off the allergic response may include:

- stopping mast cells from degranulating and pouring out allergy-creating mediators;
- using anti-IgE agents to prevent IgE antibodies from binding to mast cells, thereby blocking mediator release;
- inactivating the TH2-helper-cell mechanism that sparks the allergic response, or changing the cells into TH1 sub-types that don't stimulate IgE production (e.g., "peptide therapy" to halt the TH2 cell's production of cytokines, which stimulate IgE antibody production);
- developing other new agents to halt IgE action;
- using monoclonal antibodies directed against the TH2-helper cell's chemical messengers (cytokines), which promote IgE formation.

"Peptide therapy may well be the road to future immunotherapy," predicts the head of a Baltimore allergy clinic. "Perhaps, 50 years on, conventional immunotherapy will cease to exist. New therapies might rely on special peptides that turn off or alter the problem cells and manage to shut down IgE production and cure allergies." Another allergist predicts that "the future may see the use of T-cell modifiers (possibly self-administered) for those with allergic disorders, including asthma." In the interim, most allergy sufferers can get good to excellent relief with existing treatments.

SIX

Hay Fever

Hay fever, or seasonal allergic rhinitis – one of the most common and distressing allergies – has gone by several colorful names. In the 18th century it was called "rose cold" or "hay asthma," in the 19th century "summer catarrh," "pollenosis" or "goldenrod allergy." In the 20th century it was dubbed "hay fever" because it was particularly noticeable during the hay-pitching season. Although "hay fever" remains a popular term for this seasonal affliction – conjuring up images of sneezing, sniffling and being perpetually "stuffed up" – the disorder is not a fever, nor is it caused by hay. It has more to do with breathing in pollens from grasses, weeds and trees, and its season is not restricted to the summer months but runs from early spring through to fall.

Therefore, allergists prefer to call hay fever "seasonal allergic rhinitis" – or, more accurately, "seasonal allergic rhinoconjunctivitis" – referring to both the nasal and the eye irritation. For simplicity we'll use the terms "hay fever" and "seasonal allergic rhinitis" interchangeably in this chapter.

In the nose, inflammation of the mucous membranes that line the nasal cavity causes *rhinitis*, with itching, congestion and a clear, runny discharge. In the eyes, pollen allergens cause *conjunctivitis,* or inflammation of the *conjunctiva* (the thin membrane covering the white part of the eye and lining the eyelids), with swelling, redness, itching and teariness.

Hay fever afflicts an estimated 18 to 20 percent of North Americans at some time in their lives. Both sexes are equally affected. The disorder typically first surfaces during the teen years – from ages 12 to 16 – and may last a lifetime, although it tends to wane or vanish with increasing age. This allergy, which is apparently on the rise, brings some sufferers crowding to their physicians for relief in early spring, as trees shed their pollens; others seek advice in summer, when grasses pollinate, and still others in fall, as weeds release their pollen grains. The increase in hay-fever complaints is partly attributed to the reinforcing effects of non-allergenic irritants such as air pollutants and cigarette smoke.

Nose

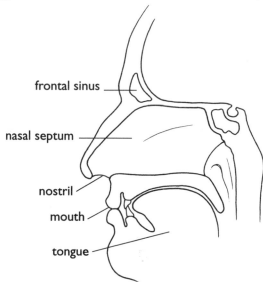

A history of hay fever

A couple of centuries ago the medical world was barely aware of hay fever. But in less than a century, seasonal allergic rhinitis has progressed from being a medical curiosity to being a very familiar disorder. The symptoms of hay fever were first medically described by an English physician, John Bostock, who in 1819 published an account of his own discomfort. Every year around early June, as Bostock recorded, he developed a "summer cold" with intense sneezing, itchy eyes and a runny nose. The condition would persist for about two months and then mysteriously vanish until the following year. Bostock never knew what caused his symptoms, but he thought they might be related to the outside temperature. Only 40 years later, in 1859, did another English physician and hay-fever sufferer, Charles Blackley, identify the cause of "summer colds." Blackley collected grass pollens all summer long; then he waited until winter, when his symptoms subsided, and inhaled a few of the pollen grains up his nose. The paroxysms of sneezing that followed tidily proved that grass pollens caused the disorder. Subsequently, Dr. Blackley spent years experimenting with different pollens. He found that as little as 0.0016 mg of pollen inhaled every 24 hours could bring on mild symptoms. He also developed a skin test for diagnosing the allergy – a test still in use today. Putting a little pollen into skin pricks on his legs made them itch, swell and develop a red patch where the pollen had been applied, clearly demonstrating a pollen sensitivity or allergic reaction.

The Main Cause – Seasonal Pollens

Seasonal allergic rhinitis is an IgE-mediated or type I allergy caused by outdoor airborne allergens, mostly pollens and molds (fungi) that are only around at certain seasons. Pollens – the microscopic male reproductive cells of many flowering plants – are the airborne allergens most commonly responsible. People with seasonal allergic rhinitis are "hypersensitive" (allergic) to one or more pollens of trees, grasses or weeds.

Not all pollens act as human allergens. Those most likely to do so come from wind-pollinated plants such as grasses, weeds and certain trees (for instance, oak and birch) that release vast quantities of light, dry pollen that can travel far and wide through the air, to make sure some grains reach their targets (female plants) and assure propagation of the species. On the whole, the more a certain pollen is around and the more of it is inhaled, the greater the likelihood of an allergy-prone person becoming sensitized to that particular pollen.

Hay fever hits during various months, depending on the type of plant someone is allergic to and when its pollen is most abundant. In North America, the pollens that generally cause rhinitis from March to late May come from trees. By June the trees have settled down but it's pollination time for summer grasses. From mid-August to October, allergies are due to weeds such as ragweed and ragwort, and the discomfort usually lasts until the first frost. The pollen season tends to start earlier in the Pacific area – in late February or early March – than in central regions, where it begins in early April; it appears still later in the Atlantic region.

Ragweed and Its Pollen

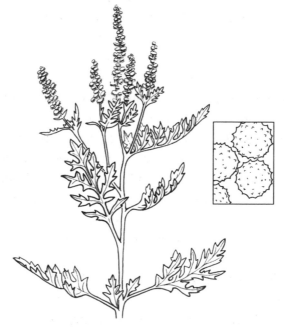

Ragweed, a grayish or yellow flowering weed, is found in many areas of North America. A single ragweed plant can spew out billions of pollen particles – to the dismay of ragweed-allergic people. In Canada, the so-called ragweed corridor extends from Windsor, Ontario, to Quebec City, where the weed grows in profusion. There is no ragweed in Newfoundland and little in the Canadian Prairies or British Columbia, except for an area around Winnipeg. The western states of the U.S. generally have less ragweed pollen than the east – for instance, there is little in Nevada and Montana. But some western states, including California, have western ragweed species that cause hay fever. There is no ragweed-free U.S. state or region.

It won't necessarily help to move away from the land of ragweed, birch and oak – studies of immigrants suggest that it often takes people only a couple of years to become sensitized to new pollens. As a service to those who are pollen-allergic, some hospitals, health units and radio stations issue daily "pollen counts," but they refer to the previous day's tally and don't necessarily predict the level of the coming day. On the whole, cool, calm or rainy days reduce the allergic discomfort; cool weather diminishes pollination, and wetness makes pollen sticky and less easily airborne. By contrast, windy weather and hot sunny days increase pollen counts.

Many people think they are allergic to various flowers, but in fact most flowers have heavy, sticky pollens that aren't windborne but are carried from plant to plant by birds, bees and other insects, or fall straight to the ground, and so do not generally cause allergic misery. However, some flower pollens can trigger rhinitis if brought into the house.

Molds Can Also Cause Hay Fever

Some seasonal rhinitis sufferers are allergic to molds and their spores, which permeate the air in moist, warm weather. Molds abound in damp climates but are sparse in deserts and drier areas. They are especially common on the shores of rivers and lakes, and grow outdoors on rotting wood, grass clippings, piles of leaves, harvested grain and other crops (for instance, corn and tomatoes), and in compost heaps. They may be abundant under the ivy growing on houses, and under other outdoor creeping plants. Indoors, they thrive in damp basements, old wallpaper and uncleaned ducts and refrigerator pans, and on clothes in poorly ventilated cupboards. Being hardier than pollens, molds and their spores can survive far colder temperatures and can create year-round allergies if dispersed from stored grain, straw and other produce.

The Christmas tree allergy that afflicts some people may be caused by molds or pollens, if these allergens stay attached to the tree after it has been cut and stored in the cold. Once the tree is indoors at the yuletide season, the warm air helps release the offending allergens that cause "Christmas season" allergic symtoms.

Typical Symptoms of Seasonal Allergic Rhinitis

Among the most striking and well-known symptoms of hay fever are the paroxysms of explosive sneezing – with 10, 20 or more sneezes in swift succession – and the stuffy nose, watery nasal discharge (possibly also an annoying post-nasal drip) and puffy, red, itchy eyes. Equally or even more irritating is the intense itching of the mouth and nose – responsible for the so-called allergic salute of rubbing the nose to relieve the itch. Congestion in the eustachian tubes can give an annoying sense of ear pressure, earache, a cracking or popping sound or muffled hearing, and can lead to ear infections.

Not surprisingly, contact-lens wearers find the swelling and itching in the eyes especially troublesome, with a gritty, dry, burning sensation that makes it hard for them to keep their

---

How do pollens trigger rhinitis?

Seasonal allergic rhinitis is an IgE-mediated problem. When the airborne allergen, such as a pollen grain or mold spore, lands on or penetrates the mucous membranes lining the human nose, throat, mouth or eyes, IgE antibodies are formed against the allergen and bind to it, stimulating release of mediators such as histamine from mast cells in the mucous membranes. The mediators produce the allergic response – the itching, sneezing, swelling, redness, runny nose and irritated, weepy eyes. There may also be a late-phase reaction some hours later, with increased inflammation and swelling. If allergen exposure is frequent, the reaction seems to be non-stop and continuous.

---

contacts in. The irritation often makes their eyes bloodshot and excessively weepy.

Seasonal rhinitis affects several parts of the body:

- *the nose* – with congestion, sneezing, itching, soreness and inflamed mucous membranes;
- *the sinuses* – which can become inflamed, blocked and painful, perhaps with headaches and sleep disturbance;
- *the eyes* – with conjunctivitis and itchiness, redness, swelling and tearing, and perhaps allergic "shiners" – dark swollen circles under and around the eyes;
- *the throat* – with "pharyngitis," an itchy red soreness, perhaps causing a cough;
- *the ears* – sometimes with blocked eustachian tubes, discomfort, infection, even temporary deafness.

The symptoms may worsen with high pollen counts, through rubbing to relieve the itch and from exposure to humidity and air pollution – smoke, perfume, chemicals and other irritants – although these are not themselves allergens.

Complications of seasonal allergic rhinitis include a hoarse voice, disturbed sleep (from the nasal stuffiness and general discomfort), ear problems (such as secondary bacterial

Common North American windborne allergens

Tree pollen
- white or silver birch
- western red cedar
- oak
- maple
- ash
- sycamore
- walnut
- mulberry
- poplar

Grass pollen
- orchard grass
- timothy
- Kentucky bluegrass
- perennial ryegrass
- june grass
- quack grass

Weed pollen
- ragweed
- artemisia species (mugworts, wormwoods, sagebrushes)
- stinging nettles
- English plantain
- lamb's quarters, goosefoot

Molds
- alternaria
- cladosporium
- aspergillus
- penicillium (mildew)

infections) and chronic mouth-breathing – which in turn leads to snoring and sleep apnea (momentary breathing stoppage), sinusitis and possibly adenoid problems. The chronic sinusitis that often results from seasonal rhinitis – with congestion in the four pairs of sinuses behind the nose and cheekbones – can lead to sensations of pressure behind the eyes, and intense headaches. Sinus headaches are typically worst in the mornings, after an overnight buildup of congestion. Congested sinuses easily develop bacterial infections – signaled by a change from the clear, runny hay-fever discharge to a thick yellow or yellow-green secretion.

Hay Fever *Can* Be Treated

During the tree-pollinating season, 34-year-old Margot, who has a birch-pollen allergy, would begin to sneeze as soon as she awakened. Her sneezing was not the light sneeze of a cold, but bursts of violent sneezes that seemed to go on forever. The worst of the sneezing was usually over by breakfast time, but Margot's nose stayed itchy and runny all day long, and got red and sore from the constant blowing. The nasal symptoms were bad enough, but Margot found her eyes still more bothersome – they were itchy, weepy, red and sore – and her ears felt "full to bursting." Her symptoms, which persisted for three to four weeks each spring, were incapacitating and exhausting. She couldn't work properly and was tired and bad-tempered.

Although appropriate medication could have helped to relieve Margot's discomfort, she refused to take drugs, trying to get by with showers to rinse off the pollen, and cool compresses for her eyes. Finally her family physician persuaded her to try some antihistamine tablets, a corticosteroid nasal spray and appropriate eyedrops, and now she no longer dreads spring each year.

Who's Most Prone to Seasonal Allergic Rhinitis?

During the 1800s, at the time of Blackley and Bostock, hay fever was considered a rare disorder. Today, however – either because it has truly increased, or because it is being better diagnosed – it has become a common chronic disorder, affecting roughly one in five North Americans. It is thought to have a hereditary component, as hay fever occurs more often when one or both parents are also sufferers, or have other allergies. Although the condition often worsens in early adulthood, it tends to diminish in middle to old age, as the immune system becomes less responsive.

Take as an example 52-year-old Laura, who has suffered from hay fever twice a year ever since she was a teenager. For Laura it was like having a prolonged bad cold every year, sneezing, sniffling and feeling miserable, with the added torment of intense itchiness in the nose and eyes. The inflammation often led to blocked sinuses, which sometimes became infected and caused terrible headaches. She remembers watching her friends enjoying springtime activities: sitting in the sun, walking in the park, playing baseball. But for Laura the month of May was a month of hiding from the spring pollens, shut up in her house with the windows closed and the air-conditioner on. She felt exhausted and stuffed up each year when school exams were on, and found it hard to concentrate. The end of summer was as bad or worse. In late August, when the ragweed began to pollinate, Laura went back indoors as her only escape. But as she got older her hay fever decreased, and by her mid-40s she wasn't as bothered by her symptoms. Now Laura doesn't even notice the pollen season.

Making the Diagnosis

A diagnosis of hay fever is often quite straightforward. It starts with a detailed history to find out the exact symptoms, when they began, and whether anyone else in the family is similarly affected. Allergic rhinitis symptoms can mimic other disorders, such as nasal polyps, asthma, enlarged adenoids and viral or bacterial infections, so the physician must make sure it's a seasonal allergy that's causing the distress. Family history also helps with diagnosis, as many people with hay fever have relatives who suffer from allergies or have asthma. The seasonal nature of the symptoms is a telltale clue that the condition may be a pollen or mold allergy. Another clue is the fact that symptoms are worst in the morning, when plants pollinate most abundantly and the air is laden with pollen. Those who are allergic to molds may find their symptoms most severe in damp weather, when these fungi produce spores.

Physical examination of the nose, throat and mouth helps confirm the diagnosis. The nasal lining membranes of those with allergic rhinitis tend to be paler in color than in someone with a cold or other infection – who may have angry red mucosal tissue – and the discharge is clear and runny rather than thick and yellowish as with viral or bacterial nose infections. Testing a smear (sample) of the nasal secretions may reveal elevated IgE antibodies and the presence of eosinophils (granular white blood cells that increase greatly with some allergies). Usually a good medical exam and a thorough history suffice to establish a diagnosis of seasonal allergic rhinitis.

To confirm the suspected pollen or seasonal mold allergy and identify the specific agents responsible, physicians may do various skin and blood tests (see Chapter Four). Pinpointing the allergens involved is essential for effective therapy.

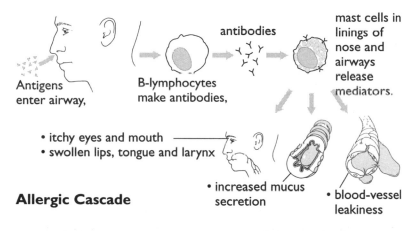

mast cells in linings of nose and airways release mediators.

antibodies

Antigens enter airway,

B-lymphocytes make antibodies,

• itchy eyes and mouth
• swollen lips, tongue and larynx

Allergic Cascade

• increased mucus secretion

• blood-vessel leakiness

Treatment: Reducing the Distress

As with all allergies, avoidance is the number-one treatment strategy. Knowing which pollens or molds are the culprits can help you reduce your exposure. If it's not possible to avoid the provocative agents, there are now plenty of anti-allergy medications to choose from.

The medications that most effectively relieve or quench seasonal allergic rhinitis include antihistamines, corticosteroids and decongestants. Remember that it's a good idea to start on the recommended medications at the onset of the triggering pollen season, not to wait until symptoms worsen. Many people suffer needlessly because they buy over-the-counter medications that are not necessarily best for their particular allergy. People who self-medicate can become frustrated if the medications don't seem to work, or produce unexpected side-effects. Advice from an allergist can be most helpful in selecting the right product, and in sorting through the myriad anti-allergy preparations. Many allergy medications are available both topically, as nasal sprays or eyedrops, and in pill form.

Types of Remedies
Hay-fever remedies include
- inhaled corticosteroid sprays
- antihistamines (as tablets, capsules, drops, sprays or syrups)
- decongestants (as tablets or sprays)
- mast-cell stabilizers (such as cromolyn) – as sprays or drops
- pollen desensitization injections (immunotherapy)

Treatment of seasonal allergic rhinitis is "customized" to the person's symptoms and their severity, bearing in mind lifestyle and social factors. In some cases the rhinitis is mild and needs minimal therapy; it may even spontaneously remit (vanish) after a few years. In others it worsens or progresses to asthma. For those with mild "once-a-year" hay fever that lasts just a few weeks, minimal drug therapy with antihistamines may be all that's needed. For those with more severe inflammatory rhinitis, topical corticosteroids may be the answer. But if drug side-effects are bothersome and symptoms are persistently severe despite proper use of medications, immunotherapy may be considered.

Checking Out the Treatments

Corticosteroid nasal sprays – for example, dexamethasone, beclomethasone, flunisolide and fluticasone – are becoming today's most widely used and effective remedies for hay fever. Many people think of antihistamines as the chief antidote, but these days low-dose corticosteroid nasal sprays are often considered first-choice treatment. The sprays reduce the levels of allergic mediators and lessen the inflammation, but they should be started right at the beginning of the allergy season and used regularly, as they take a week or so to achieve maximum effect. Taken throughout the pollen season, corticosteroid nasal sprays have no serious adverse effects and are not absorbed into the body; they act locally. The dose is adjusted to give sufficient relief with the smallest possible amount; a once-daily dose is often enough. Minor side-effects include some nasal dryness and irritation, and possibly slight nosebleeds. Corticosteroid sprays can be used together with antihistamines for optimal relief. If steroids are to be used long term, however, the nasal passages should be examined regularly during medical checkups.

Antihistamines have long been a mainstay of allergy treatment. Generally safe, they act in 15 to 30 minutes and work for three to six hours. Since antihistamines *prevent* symptoms rather than curing them, it is best to start them at the first hint of rhinitis symptoms, rather than waiting for the discomfort to become severe, when they will not work as well. Antihistamines help relieve the sneezing, nose-watering and weeping but don't do much for the nasal stuffiness, which requires decongestants or anti-inflammatories.

Second-generation antihistamines are less sedating and cause fewer annoying side-effects than the earlier first-generation antihistamines, so have been of great benefit to countless allergy sufferers. Some of them take longer to start acting, but others – such as loratadine (Claritin) and cetirizine (Reactine) – are both nonsedating and fast-acting. As one radio host puts it: "I survive on antihistamines right through the ragweed season – from late August to the end of October."

As discussed in Chapter Five, some second-generation anti-histamines – in particular astemizole and terfenadine – can produce heart-rhythm disturbances if taken with certain antibiotics, antifungals such as ketoconazole or the ulcer remedy cimetidine.

Decongestants, many available without prescription, are agents that help to eliminate or relieve nasal stuffiness or congestion by constricting tiny blood vessels, reducing fluid accumulation and swelling. Decongestants are best taken by mouth. Oral forms include over-the-counter products such as phenyl-propanolamine, pseudoephedrine and naphazoline. They have a stimulant effect (unlike the sedating antihistamines) and tend to "perk people up," although they can also cause irritability, insomnia, nervousness, heart palpitations and dizziness. Excessive use of decongestants can raise blood pressure and cause kidney problems and heart irregularities. Consult a physician before embarking on long-term oral decongestants if you have heart or blood-pressure problems, glaucoma, a kidney disorder, prostate trouble, seizures, hyperthyroidism or any other medical disorder. Also, if you take decongestants over the long term be sure to have your blood pressure checked regularly.

Topical decongestant nasal sprays should never be used for more than five days at a time, as "drug tolerance" tends to develop; this leads to "rebound congestion" or "nasal spray addiction," also called "rhinitis medicamentosa," with more rather than less nasal stuffiness – a condition that's notoriously hard to treat or eradicate. Topical decongestant or vasoconstrictor drops can be very useful for the eyes, but again not for too long. (See Chapter Thirteen.)

Mast-cell stabilizers such as cromolyn (also called "cromo-glycate") are another class of medication that can help hay-fever sufferers, by preventing release of histamine from mast cells, curbing the inflammatory effects. Cromolyn is a very safe medication with no side-effects, suitable even for young children, but it works best as a preventive, and must be used regularly to have any impact. Some forms are also available as eyedrops.

Another nasal spray, ipratropium, can help cut down mucus production and ease the congestion; nasal saline spray (available in drugstores) may be helpful in soothing sore, crusted nasal tissues.

Experts warn that although there is a plethora of "combination" anti-allergy products on the market – containing an antihistamine, decongestant *and* painkiller or headache remedy, for instance – it's much safer and wiser to take the various drugs separately than as a mixture. Taking the medications one by one allows you to assess the dose, and gauge the drug's effectiveness and any adverse reactions that may occur.

Finding the Right Drug Takes Trial and Error

Thong has had hay fever since he arrived in North America when he was 17 years old. He coped with it as best he could, but never really managed his symptoms well. He tried older forms of over-the-counter antihistamines; they reduced the perpetual nasal itch and dripping but made him sleepy. Mostly he just sneezed and sniffled through the grass-pollen season each summer. Now 31, he is trying to finish up a doctorate and feels he can't afford to waste each summer feeling wretched. He consulted a hospital allergist, who pinpointed rye grass as the culprit and suggested Thong try one of the modern, nonsedating antihistamines. But Thong thought the medication made him somewhat dull-witted. The allergist then tried him on inhaled corticosteroids – twice daily – which seemed to do the trick. Thong finds that if he starts the medication in time – as soon as the first grass pollens begin to fly – he can make it through the summer with minimal discomfort.

Immunotherapy Is a "Long Shot"

Properly administered, immunotherapy is effective against seasonal allergic rhinitis for a small number of sufferers, provided it's geared to the specific pollens creating the symptoms. Canadian and U.S. allergy organizations recommend pollen extract injections for a minority of hay-fever sufferers: those in whom medications and avoidance have failed to bring relief, and a few people with asthma who are also allergic to dust mites and ragweed. Immunotherapy should not be used for those with autoimmune conditions, severe asthma or coronary heart disease.

Allergy injections for pollen-induced hay fever were first tried in 1911 by two American scientists who believed that

Drops and sprays for sore, itchy eyes

Oral medications sometimes fail to relieve the itchy, gritty, sticky eyes that accompany hay fever, but many allergy medications now come as eyedrops. Vasoconstrictors or "eye whiteners" such as naphazoline or oxymetazoline help decrease eye redness and swelling. Antihistamine drops such as antazoline reduce itching and a new form, levocabastine, can reduce most allergic eye symptoms. Lodoxamide and ketorolac are other eye medications suitable for short-term (one-month) use. Cromolyn also comes as eyedrops (Opticrom).

Some anti-allergy eye medications have minor side-effects such as transient stinging, and are not recommended for contact-lens wearers; you can consult an eye specialist about suitable choices. Corticosteroid eyedrops are occasionally prescribed for rhinitis sufferers, but must be taken sparingly and definitely *under medical supervision*, as they can increase the risks of cataract and glaucoma. (See also Chapter Thirteen.)

pollen produced a toxin that made people sneeze. By analogy with other therapies being developed at the time, the scientists thought that if they administered gradually increasing doses of the "poison-producing" pollen into the skin, the body would slowly adjust to it, probably by producing antitoxins to neutralize the pollen's effect. Their idea was wrong: pollen does *not* produce a toxin. But the treatment seemed to work, and the researchers found that slowly increasing the concentration of injected pollen reduced allergic sensitivity in some people, alleviating hay-fever symptoms, at least for a while.

Better-purified pollen extracts and more precise guidelines for immunotherapy have helped to make the injections worthwhile. A skin prick test must first positively identify the exact pollens to which someone is allergic. Once the suspect pollen is pinpointed, extracts are injected, weekly at first, then monthly. Immunotherapy is thought to work by stimulating a rise in non-allergy-producing antibodies (IgG antibodies) at the expense of allergy-provoking IgE antibodies, so that IgE levels fall. The concentration of the pollen extracts injected must be high enough. Over time, the injections reduce pollen sensitivity, with improvement often noticeable within six months to a year of starting the shots. Correctly administered, immunotherapy reduces symptoms to some extent in about 70 percent of people with severe hay fever. When the shots are stopped, about two-thirds remain relatively symptom-free, while the distress is lessened in others. A few people relapse entirely.

The drawback to pollen desensitization is that the technique is time-consuming and requires weekly or monthly injections for several years. Health-insurance schemes may pay for allergy injections but the patient may have to cover the cost of the pollen extracts used. Although it's rare, there is some risk of a severe reaction, such as swelling and hives, on injection, so

– again – allergy shots should only be given by properly equipped doctors, and people should remain in the physician's waiting room for 20 minutes after the treatment, for surveillance in case of side-effects.

Tips for preventing hay fever

- Avoid pollen exposure as much as possible.
- Avoid exercising outdoors during the relevant pollen season, especially when pollen counts are highest – usually from 6 a.m. to 10 a.m., or in very hot, dry or windy weather.
- Don't rake leaves or mow grass; this stirs up pollen grains.
- Wear a disposable mask when working outdoors or gardening at the height of the pollen season.
- Close windows to keep pollen out.
- Use an air-conditioner, but be sure the filters are kept clean and not allowed to collect molds, which could worsen the allergy.
- Note that car air-conditioners easily grow molds; air out your vehicle well, and don't aim the vents directly at your face.
- Shower often to help wash pollen out of your hair and off your skin.
- Avoid room fans – they're notorious for stirring up pollen and other substances.
- Keep the house cool but not cold.
- Don't hang clothes outside to dry, as they may pick up pollen.
- Keep molds down by keeping house humidity at 30 percent or less with a dehumidifier, and cleaning out mold-ridden areas – such as refrigerator and dehumidifier pans, basement corners and bathrooms – with bleach or household cleaning solution from time to time.
- Put a dehumidifier in the basement.
- Plan your vacation in a low-pollen or pollen-free area if possible.

SEVEN

Year-round Indoor Allergies

While the pollens that cause hay fever vanish with the first heavy frost, other airborne allergens are not seasonal but persist all year long. *Perennial allergic rhinitis* – a year-round allergy with symptoms similar to hay fever – is a chronic inflammatory disorder affecting the mucous membranes of the nose, eyes and upper airways. Its main symptoms are an itchy nose and palate, sneezing bouts, conjunctivitis (sore, weepy eyes) and nasal stuffiness. The nasal congestion is often worse and more distressing than with hay fever.

The airborne indoor allergens chiefly to blame for perennial rhinitis include molds (fungi and their spores), animal dander, cockroach and other insect parts, dried pollens, dust mites and their by-products and the accumulated detritus we know as "house dust." Occasionally, bacteria growing in humidifiers, or accumulated in refrigerator drip pans, clothes-dryer exhaust pipes or organic material, act as indoor allergens. Indoor plants rarely cause allergic reactions, except for *Ficus benjamina* and flowering maple.

Rhinitis from indoor allergens plagues countless people. Since urban people now spend much of their time indoors, it's an increasing problem. Swedish studies find that indoor rhinitis affects 15 percent of men and 14 percent of women; in North America about 8 to 10 percent of the population suffers from year-round rhinitis, sometimes in addition to hay fever or asthma. It affects both sexes and all races. Year-round rhinitis tends to start younger than hay fever, usually surfacing around age ten or in early adulthood, but it can strike at any age. With advancing age it tends to wane; many of the middle-aged and elderly no longer suffer from allergic rhinitis. Improved understanding of nasal physiology and how the nose functions is improving the management of this distressing disorder.

The Nose Is a Prime Target

Although conjunctivitis is sometimes the main complaint of those with allergic rhinitis – and some experts prefer to call the disorder *rhinoconjunctivitis* – the nasal symptoms are a more familiar and distinguishing feature: itching, sneezing paroxysms, swollen mucous membranes and inflammation. (Eye allergies are fully described in Chapter Thirteen.)

Allergic rhinitis disturbs the normal function of the nose – impairs its capacity to smell, and to trap and filter out harmful particles and protect the airways by the sweeping action of its little hairs or *cilia*. It obstructs the air flow and alters nasal secretions. Normally these secretions contain many different compounds, among them antibacterial agents. By interfering with the nasal secretions and causing swelling and inflammation, allergic rhinitis often leads to sinusitis (sinus infection) and increased nasal infections. Rhinitis also distorts normal voice production, giving speech a nasal tone.

Like hay fever, perennial rhinitis is an IgE-mediated immune response with detectably elevated IgE antibody levels. The triggering allergen enters the nose, attaches to IgE antibodies and

> ### Air pollutants may aggravate symptoms
>
> Perennial allergic rhinitis may be made more severe by irritants such as tobacco smoke, aerosols, strong odors, insecticides, and cooking and chemical fumes. In fact, irritants such as perfumes, certain chemicals and even light can cause nonallergic (irritant) rhinitis through mechanisms not related to the immune system. Some studies find that perennial allergic rhinitis and asthma have a confirmed link to air pollution. Other variables such as overcrowding, lack of medical care and poverty may play a role.
>
> There's considerable evidence that tobacco smoke increases the risk of indoor rhinitis and asthma. One U.S. study linked parental smoking to an increased likelihood of allergic rhinitis in children. A recent Swedish study found the incidence of indoor allergy higher than average in babies of smoking mothers. Rhinitis also tends to be worsened by colds, cooking fumes and certain chemicals (such as formaldehyde).

stimulates mast cells and basophils to liberate potent mediators. Pre-formed mediators (such as histamine) cause the immediate nasal itch and sneezing. The later release of newly synthesized mediators causes more prolonged nasal inflammation. This "late phase" reaction perpetuates the nasal distress, sustaining the rhinitis.

Identifying Perennial Allergic Rhinitis and Its Triggers

The telltale clues to allergic rhinitis are an itchy nose and palate, violent sneezing fits, a clear, runny nasal discharge and nasal stuffiness. The first step in diagnosis is a thorough medical history to exclude other disorders that can cause the same symptoms – for example, a structural nose defect or obstruction, polyps, a foreign body in the nose (most often found in children) and *irritant rhinitis* – the latter can arise from increased sympathetic nervous system (vasomotor) activity due to irritants such as alcohol, spicy food, fragrances, extreme cold, even bright light or emotional distress. In such cases, sneezing is less common. Some diseases – such as hypothyroidism (too little thyroid hormone) or diabetes – can cause rhinitis, and certain medications (such as diuretics and drugs to lower blood pressure) may produce nasal congestion.

The physical examination will include a careful look at the head, neck, nose, eyes and chest. The examination may reveal the bluish, unhealthy-looking, swollen nasal membranes typical of allergic rhinitis. (Irritant rhinitis and infections produce a deep red nasal lining.) The eyes may be sore and weepy with dark circles ("allergic shiners") under them. The sinuses may be blocked, and polyps may be detected in the nasal passages. Mouth-breathing is common because of the congested nose.

Most perennial allergic rhinitis can be traced to a few common indoor allergens. Someone who starts to weep and sneeze as soon as a cat enters the room is clearly allergic to cats. Someone who develops symptoms when staying in a damp basement is likely allergic to molds. But sometimes the cause is obscure. For example, a person who has lived for many years with a dog in the house may have continual minor nasal stuffiness without knowing that the pet is to blame. A few people develop sensitivity to rare allergens; in a Swiss study, bed quilts filled with wild silk from China caused allergic asthma. Because houseplant allergies are rare, they may easily be overlooked as a source of the problem. Chemicals known to cause indoor rhinitis include anhydrides in plastic materials, metal salts, ethylene diamine in paint finishes and some modern furnishings.

Skin prick tests may be done with extracts of molds, cockroach, animal dander, pollens and dust mite to try to confirm the diagnosis and determine what's precipitating the symptoms. Nasal provocation tests may be tried for elusive cases: a little of the allergen extract is instilled into the nose to see if symptoms appear. A RAST (blood) test is of limited value for indoor allergens.

Non-allergic Causes of Rhinitis

Rhinitis can arise from many causes other than IgE-mediated allergy. Take for example Andrew, who goes into paroxysms of sneezing whenever he steps into bright sunlight, especially from a darkened room. Or Emily, who in her second trimester of pregnancy began to suffer symptoms of rhinitis. Or Jason, who has chronic nasal congestion, sleeps with his mouth open, snores loudly and frequently awakens from his sleep. Each of these three people thought the cause of the problem was an allergy. But on medical investigation each turned out to have another condition that mimics some aspects of allergic rhinitis. Andrew suffers from an unusual type of *vasomotor rhinitis* – a reaction triggered by a number of causes, including bright sunlight. Emily has *hormonal rhinitis* – a transient condition brought on by increased hormone levels during pregnancy. Jason was found to have enlarged adenoids, which not only caused his snoring but also disturbed his sleep, and required surgery.

Some Causes of Non-allergic Rhinitis
- *Vasomotor or irritant rhinitis* – with watery, runny nose and nasal congestion, provoked by irritants such as smoke, light, temperature changes, spicy foods and emotional upsets.
- *Bacterial infections leading to sinusitis* – with chronic nasal congestion, bad breath and a cough (often following an infection of the upper respiratory tract).
- *Hormone changes* – leading to nasal congestion and sneezing – brought on by diabetes, thyroid imbalance or an increase in certain hormones during pregnancy.

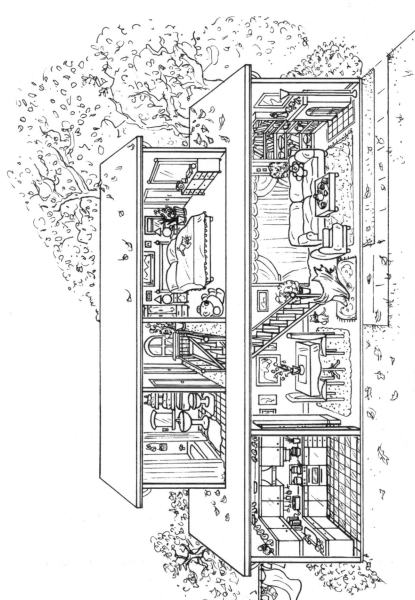

Where Allergies Lurk

Questions the allergist may ask

- Do the symptoms improve or vanish when you are out of the house or away on holiday?
- Do your sisters and brothers or parents have similar problems? (Sometimes similar environmental triggers bring on symptoms in several family members.)
- Are your symptoms worse in the morning? (Bedrooms that collect dust – and dust mites – can be a source of allergic symptoms that worsen overnight but clear up during the day.)
- Do your symptoms get worse in certain parts of the house? (Allergens vary in quantity from room to room. Kitchens are more likely to harbor cockroach allergens, while molds are most likely to inhabit damp basements or bathrooms.)
- Has a new pet come into your house?

- *Structural abnormalities* such as a deviated nasal septum, nasal polyps, enlarged adenoids, nasal tumors.
- *Rhinitis medicamentosa* – an angry, red nasal inflammation and severe congestion due to a rebound effect from repetitive use of topical decongestant nasal sprays. Used for more than five to seven days, topical nasal decongestants can worsen rather than relieve nasal stuffiness; this condition is hard to reverse and may even require a short course of oral corticosteroids.

Possible Complications of Allergic Rhinitis

Untreated rhinitis often leads to nasal polyps and chronic sinusitis. Nasal polyps are smooth, pear-shaped, translucent, gelatinous outgrowths of the nasal lining, most usual after age 40 or so, and rare in children and adolescents. They arise from prolonged nasal swelling, inflammation and irritation and can increase the risk of sinusitis. Polyps have long been linked to indoor allergies and asthma. Treatment is with corticosteroid nasal sprays, which effectively shrink the polyps. (Surgical removal is now rarely done because the polyps so often recur.)

Sinusitis is a chronic bacterial infection of the sinuses in which the mucus stagnates and becomes infected. It typically occurs after a head cold, when symptoms fail to clear in a couple of weeks, and is heralded by a thick yellowish-green discharge, a dull headache and sharp pain in the jaw and cheeks. The blocked sinuses can also cause earache. Treatment is with painkillers, decongestants to clear the sinuses, corticosteroids to reduce the inflammation and antibiotics to get rid of the bacterial infection. Steam and saline sprays may also help to clear the nasal congestion.

Taking a Closer Look at Indoor Allergens

Dust Components

Not surprisingly, dust is a prime allergy-causer, as it's all around and easily airborne. Besides rhinitis, dust components often aggravate asthma and eczema (although the link between eczema and dust mites is not yet fully established). People often loosely say they're "allergic to dust" because they have sneezing attacks in dusty rooms, but not all dust constituents cause allergies. Allergies stem from specific components – pollens, the feces of dust mites and insect parts.

Animal Dander

With the increasing popularity of pets, animal allergies are said to affect up to 20 percent of the North American population – especially cat and dog allergies. Many of those affected also have asthma. Animal handlers tend to have allergies to the species they most frequently deal with. Farm workers typically suffer from horse, cow, pig or sheep allergies.

All animals – even birds – can cause allergies, because of potent allergens in their saliva or on their coats or feathers. The best-studied animal allergen is from cats – one of the most allergy-provoking animals. Cat allergies are becoming a major

Nasal Polyps

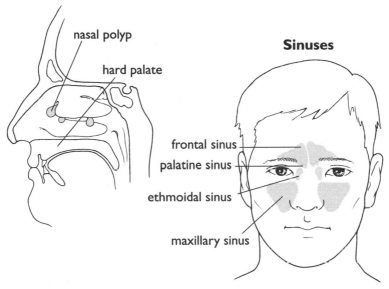

nasal polyp

hard palate

Sinuses

frontal sinus

palatine sinus

ethmoidal sinus

maxillary sinus

North American problem, given that 28 percent of households have at least one cat. The allergic reaction is caused not by the whole animal, or even by cat saliva, but by certain molecules in the animal's saliva, skin and urine. (Cat dander is a mixture of saliva and skin flakes.) The precise compounds responsible for triggering the allergic response are slowly being identified. The major identified cat allergen is fel d I – an acidic glycoprotein that's present in the cat hair, saliva and skin; concentrations are greatest at the hair root but are distributed by the animal's grooming. Male cats have higher levels than females. When dried out, these molecules float on airborne dust particles and enter the nose and eyes, causing nasal, eye and respiratory symptoms. Classrooms and catless places may contain cat allergens brought in on clothes or shoes.

The cat-dander allergen clings tenaciously to carpets, furniture and walls, and can linger for months after a cat has left the premises. Aggressive cleaning may speed up cat-allergen removal, but steam-cleaning doesn't help. Human beings can carry the allergen around on their clothes, spreading it from house to house and to school and work settings. No breed of cat is more allergy-provoking than another, although individual cats vary. (Lions and tigers also have fel d I antigens.)

The dog allergen, can f I, is found in the saliva of all breeds, from curly-haired Airedales to short-haired boxers or long-haired Afghans. Like the cat allergen, can f I persists in the environment after a dog is long gone, and can be carried about on the clothes of dog owners, causing allergic distress even when there is no dog in the vicinity. Allergies to dogs are less common than cat allergies.

According to popular belief (and some dog lovers), certain breeds such as poodles, Portuguese water dogs and wheaten terriers are "non-allergenic." However, one allergist emphasizes that "all dogs can cause allergies and no breed is non-allergenic." She has seen many a sniffing and sneezing poodle owner who had to part with a beloved pet.

Rodents, such as hamsters, guinea pigs, gerbils, mice, rats and rabbits, are all known allergy-causers. Surveys of people who work with small animals in laboratories find that 10 to 15 percent have some allergic sensitivity, and these animals also cause allergies when kept as pets. The allergen is found in the urine of mice, rats and guinea pigs, and in the saliva and on the fur of rabbits. Rodent allergy is a major problem in workers exposed to laboratory animals. Mouse and rat proteins in air filters, pipes and urban houses are blamed for some allergies in the general population.

Horse allergy is caused by the horse allergens equ c I, II, III. Horse allergies are now less common than before, as horses are no longer used to work in the streets, nor do we use horsehair furniture, blankets, mattresses and felts as much as we once did. Some 10 to 12 percent of allergic people have positive skin reactions to horse allergens. People who react to horses may also react to mules, donkeys and zebras.

Birds such as canaries, budgies and pigeons are known to cause allergies; they are more commonly a problem in those who work in bird-breeding and farming. People allergic to birds can eat chicken and eggs without reacting, but may react to feathers in down comforters, duvets, beds, pillows and sleeping bags – although such reactions may also be caused by dust mites. Birds can also provoke allergies in those who process eggs – about 10 percent of egg-workers develop asthma blamed on allergies to avian proteins. As well, birds can cause a pneumonia-like condition called *hypersensitivity pneumonitis.*

Insect Parts

Although the ground-up parts of all sorts of insects have been identified as major allergy-causers – including moths, beetles, flies and locusts, to name a few – cockroaches are the most common culprits in urban North America. One Chicago study found that 60 percent of asthma sufferers at an allergy clinic were sensitized to cockroaches. A recent University of Toronto study found 6 percent of patients attending a local allergy clinic were cockroach-sensitive. Children living in inner-city cockroach-infested apartments are at special risk. Suburban children are less likely to have cockroach allergies.

Houseplants

Considering the havoc wrought by outdoor tree pollens in spring, it's surprising how few indoor plants reportedly cause allergies. One likely explanation is that most indoor plants are leafy green rather than flowering types and pollinate less profusely. *Ficus benjamina* (weeping fig), a popular indoor tree, has been reported to cause eye allergies. The nectar of the *Abutilon striatum* (flowering maple) can trigger asthma.

Molds

Molds (fungi) thrive in carpets, plastic, wastebins, books, magazines and bedding. Some forms feed on the sulfur in concrete, or on paint or glue. Molds produce spores that are well known to trigger wheezing and other respiratory discomfort. They grow best in humid conditions, and indoor types also prefer the dark. Key trouble spots include damp basements, shower stalls, gratings, bathrooms and moist carpeting or furnishings. Outdoor fungi grow best in shaded areas, organic debris and unkempt property. Some molds used to produce wines, cheeses and other foods can also cause allergies; wine-makers and cheese-makers are apt to get mold allergies.

The Mighty Dust Mite

Scientists have known since early this century that house dust triggers allergic symptoms, but they originally thought this was because of the animal dander, insect parts and other collected debris it contains. Only in 1967 did researchers in The Netherlands show that the major cause of IgE reactivity in dust-sensitive people is the dust mite, a tiny arthropod that lives in house dust. In fact, it's not the mite itself that enters human airways but fragments of its feces – light enough to be airborne and small enough to penetrate the mucous membranes of the nose and eyes. (Mite feces are about the size of tiny pollen grains, and mite allergens include several proteins, der p I, II and III.) Ground-up mite parts can also be potent sensitizers. Dust-mite sensitization depends on the concentration of mites and their feces; allergic reactions are less likely at lower concentrations. Recent studies show that mite-sensitization often occurs in infancy, and also show an alarming increase in dust-mite allergies, especially among children in poor neighborhoods and among urban U.S. blacks. The allergen has been implicated in serious asthma and a few deaths.

Dust Mite

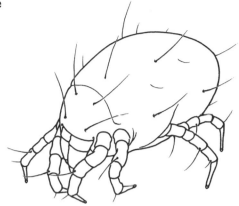

The dust mite is an otherwise harmless, sightless, wingless, eight-legged creature of the spider family, measuring about 0.3 mm long (about a hundredth of an inch), visible only under the microscope. Its scientific name, *Dermatophagoides pteronyssinus* ("skin eating"), denotes the fact that mites eat and live on the skin scales of people and other animals.

Dust mites cannot drink, but they absorb water from the air via special moisture attractants in their leg joints. Since they need moisture to survive, they do best in damp, humid environments (particularly basements). They thrive in roughly the same temperature and humidity conditions that suit humans – around 70°F (21°C) and 22 to 26 percent humidity. The lower the temperature and humidity, the likelier it is that the mites will shrivel up and die. Freezing kills them, but their droppings may continue to trigger symptoms.

Mites are especially numerous in mattresses, carpets and pillows, which are all rich in human skin sheddings; of 47 known species, 11 have been identified in mattresses and bedding. One bed may house 200 million mites. To fight them, completely enclose mattresses and pillows in airtight plastic or vinyl cases, or in special covers that are now readily available. They can't get through thick plastic, so covering mattresses and box springs keeps them out. A cheaper alternative is to wrap pillows in thick plastic garbage bags, and mattresses in strong plastic sheeting available from hardware stores. The wrapping must be well sealed with tape. Putting a towel liner between the plastic-wrapped pillow and the pillowcase, and using a cotton blanket as an undersheet, will make the pillows and mattress less slippery. Damp-wipe the mattress cover every two weeks. Wash all bedding frequently in very hot water, and dry at a hot setting.

Cockroaches

To combat cockroaches, keep the kitchen clean and don't leave food out in other rooms. Seal off insect-entry points into the home. Cover all food and dispose of garbage promptly. If roaches appear, use roach-killer.

Managing a Pet Allergy

Common sense dictates that if someone has severe allergic symptoms or asthma brought on by a pet, it's best to steer clear of the animal or get rid of it. But disposing of a family pet can be heart-rending and divisive for the entire family, and especially hard on a child whose allergy may be responsible for the discord. It's hardly surprising that many people – even those with severe allergies – refuse to part with a beloved animal.

One veterinarian suggests, "Wash the cat" – a controversial approach! Rinsing or swabbing down a cat with warm water, contrary to popular opinion, does not get rid of a considerable amount of cat allergen. Experts vary in their recommendations as to whether, how and how often to wash a cat. One strategy is to gently wash the cat with pet shampoo once a week for three or four weeks and then cut back to once a month or less, watching whether the allergic symptoms decrease. Better yet, have someone else wash the cat. Those with a dog allergy can do likewise and wash the dog once a week – probably less of a hassle than washing a cat!

Occasionally, pet tolerance develops and the allergic person gets used to the mild symptoms, so that pet and owner can harmoniously coexist. In intermediate situations, the risks and benefits of keeping the animal can be evaluated. Many strategies have been worked out to allow people to keep a pet despite the problems it causes. Nevertheless, keeping a pet in a home where someone is severely allergic means continual use of allergy medications, with their attendant expense and side-effects. On the other hand, disposing of a pet can be traumatic and will not relieve other allergies – such as a dust-mite or pollen allergy. Sometimes people who cannot bear to part with their pet demand allergy shots to reduce the discomfort. Allergists may hesitate to give injections to people who could get rid of the cause – mainly because of the expense, time and inconvenience of immunotherapy – but some agree to administer shots if medication and house-cleaning fail to clear the symptoms.

Joanna, aged 20, is a cat lover who is severely allergic to cats. She recently moved into a student household with two furry and affectionate cats who were irresistible to play with. At first she developed red, weepy eyes, sneezing and other symptoms whenever she was in close contact with the cats. After a few weeks, however, the allergic symptoms became less troublesome; she developed some tolerance and was able to live with the cats quite happily. By contrast, Jane, who was cat-allergic and also sensitive to dust and molds, came to share the same house and found her allergies worsened. As well as being full of cat dander, the house was old and dusty. Within a few weeks of moving in, Jane found that her nasal symptoms became increasingly severe; her eyes were always itchy and she felt utterly miserable. Medications such as antihista-mines and decongestants didn't help. Keeping the cats out of her bedroom wasn't much help either. Finally she moved into a modern apartment with good ventilation, hardwood floors and air-conditioning. Jane keeps her apartment clean and dust-free. Instead of a cat she keeps a couple of goldfish, and her symptoms have gone. But she still gets sniffly and red-eyed when she goes to visit any household with cats.

Treating Year-round Allergic Rhinitis

Once the diagnosis is confirmed and the allergen is identified, the next step is managing the situation. Three strategies help control perennial rhinitis: environmental control, or avoiding the offensive allergens; use of appropriate medications; and immunotherapy, in a few instances. As with all allergies, avoid-ance is the key. Although some allergens cannot be entirely avoided, various measures can reduce the level of allergens in your home (see below).

Pharmacotherapy is the next step, with judicious use of the many medications available. First choice among the available drugs are antihistamines. Although some physicians believe the usefulness of antihistamines wears off with time, studies do not show that such tolerance develops; they remain excellent antidotes against the dripping nose, sneezing and itching, but not the nasal congestion.

To reduce congestion, you can use decongestant tablets such as pseudoephedrine or propanolamine – in recommended doses, as an excess can cause jitteriness and insomnia. Corti-costeroid nasal sprays reduce local inflammation, constrict blood vessels and reduce the swelling.

The best idea is to use an integrated course of medications planned by your physician, as no one drug will do the trick. Mast-cell stabilizers such as cromolyn or nedocromil are good for prevention of symptoms, if taken before exposure – as when a cat-allergic person must visit a cat-owning relative. (See Chapter Five for a full rundown of anti-allergy medications.)

Immunotherapy (allergen injections) may be tried for perennial allergic rhinitis that has not responded to careful avoidance and drug treatment. It can be useful for cat, mold and dust-mite allergies.

Future Therapies

Already, drugs that combat the action of specific mediators are being developed. As well, vaccines of specific allergens, designed to interrupt the immune process, are being tested in the U.S. and Canada and have so far been found safe and effective. Over the next few years vaccines against cat protein, ragweed, pollen, dust-mite and other indoor allergens will likely be developed.

Allergy-Proofing Your Home

One expert remarks that "if only people had the will and the means, allergen avoidance is quite easy. Often, all that's needed to stop allergy symptoms is an air-conditioned, low-humidity home, with polished wooden floors, leather or wooden furniture, a simple bedroom with a covered mattress, no clutter, no carpets and no pets allowed in the bedroom. Thick carpets, padded chairs and sofas are allergen reservoirs. If possible, windows that open and allow good ventilation are a plus."

Ripping up the carpet and polishing the floor can eliminate 98 percent of dust mites. But for those who prefer not to throw out their carpets, common mite-killing compounds (acaricides) such as benzyl benzoate, available as a powder, foam or liquid, may eradicate enough mites to reduce the symptoms. Neither foam nor liquid mite-killers have proven fully effective, according to one expert, and the powder only works if properly applied. It should be brushed into the carpet, left overnight and then brushed in again before vacuuming. If this is done well, its cleaning effect can last three months. Tannic acid (a 3 percent solution) sprayed onto a just-cleaned carpet can also be effective against dust-mite allergens. The spray guards against mites for six weeks to two months. Products that kill dust mites and protect the home can be found at the pharmacy or ordered from mail-order catalogs, and they need to be used regularly.

Scrupulous Cleaning Also Helps

Cockroaches and mites are notoriously hard to vanquish. The goal is to arrange furniture and upholstery so that it can be kept as free of mold and dust as possible. Carpets contain 100 times more dust than wood or tiles, so they should be removed wherever feasible. Air-conditioners and dehumidifiers can reduce the humidity to make the environment less dust-friendly. In general, the best strategy is to start in the bedroom, and if necessary follow with allergen-removal in the rest of the house. Bedrooms should be cleared of stuffed furniture, carpets, dust-attracting curtains, blinds and knick-knacks.

Vacuuming alone removes dust particles but *not* dust mites or molds. For efficient vacuuming, use double-layer bags or additional filters such as HEPA (high-efficiency particulate air) in the vacuum cleaner; cheap bags allow dust leakage. Consider renting a HEPA air filter for a few months and see if it works in reducing symptoms; many allergists doubt their usefulness. To remove molds, swab surfaces in humid areas with bleach from time to time. (See the table of allergen-removing tactics below.)

While stringent cleaning measures certainly reduce allergen levels, it's not clear whether less draconian methods also help. Some measures are very tiring, mind-occupying and time-consuming, and allergy experts disagree about just how much is enough. They warn that environmental control is not the cure for all allergies, and that results are highly variable. Some symptoms may linger even after scrupulous cleaning, vacuuming, refurnishing and renovating efforts. Many people still need medications to achieve relief. Probably moderation is the answer – keep the home dust-free, but don't be obsessive about it.

Control House Temperature and Humidity
Since dust mites thrive best at temperatures above 77°F (25°C), the temperature in the house should be kept between 68 and 71°F (20 and 21°C). Reduce humidity in damp areas by using a dehumidifier set between 25 and 30 percent, as dust mites cannot live at low levels of humidity.

There is no ideal heating system for the allergic person. Forced-air heating is probably the least expensive option, but furnace filters must be cleaned weekly and replaced monthly during the heating season. Baseboard electrical heaters and hot-water radiators are not very effective at maintaining a uniform temperature throughout the room, and they tend to collect dust so they need to be cleaned often. Heat pumps may be very energy-efficient but they constantly bring in outside air laden with pollens and other irritants. All ductwork should be occasionally vacuumed by a professional furnace-cleaning firm so dust and dust mites are not recirculated.

Vents in the bedroom may be covered with a piece of standard furnace filter to block out dust, and beds should not be placed in line with the ducts. Avoid using kerosene heaters and wood or coal stoves, as they produce smoke, carbon monoxide, sulfur dioxide and other gases that can be irritating. For air cooling, both central and portable air-conditioners help, as they make conditions more comfortable indoors when doors

The lowdown on air cleaners

Despite advertising promises, portable air cleaners or filtering devices do not effectively remove particles from the air. All other dust-reducing procedures should be tried first, because no filter can take the place of effective cleaning. Mite antigens are heavy and fall quickly, so cleaning – rather than filters – is the most effective way to reduce them. "The only worthwhile cleaners," explains one indoor air expert, "are the high-efficiency particulate air, or HEPA, filters. To work effectively, filters should be replaced as advised by the manufacturer. The disadvantage of these units is that they're expensive. There's no point buying a small, desktop air cleaner, as it will do little more than freshen the room. Larger units with mechanical filters remove only large particles that don't create allergy problems anyway." Place portable HEPA filters only on clean, bare floors (never on rugs). An electrostatic filter can remove smaller airborne particles, but in the process it releases ozone as a by-product, which is an irritant for many allergic people. Negative-ion machines have no proven value for people with allergies.

and windows are closed to keep out allergens. Although they don't clean air effectively, as they operate only intermittently, they are helpful in reducing humidity.

Ways to Control Mold Growth

- Wash surfaces such as window ledges and shower stalls with mold-killing household cleaner or chlorine bleach at least every three months. (As these cleaners release irritating fumes, rinse well and air the room afterwards.)
- Use dehumidifiers and clean them frequently.
- Clean ventilation equipment and replace filters often in furnaces, air-conditioners and dehumidifiers.
- Disinfect vaporizers before using, and often during the season of use.
- Cover soil of houseplants with plastic wrap, or add a mold-inhibiting solution (available at nurseries) to the soil.
- Keep aquariums small and out of bedrooms.

- Cover the ground in crawl spaces with black polyethylene sheets.
- Install drains that effectively remove standing water.
- Use exhaust fans, vented to the outside, after bathing or when cooking or laundering, to remove water vapor.
- Use mold-resistant paint on unfinished basement walls.
- Leave a low-wattage lightbulb on as a heat source in damp closets, or store some hygroscopic (water-absorbing) crystals on the top shelf, out of children's reach.
- Increase sunlight in the garden by trimming or cutting down trees and shrubs.

A Summary of How to Cope with Indoor Allergens

- Keep rooms well ventilated.
- "Damp dust" regularly; try using a specially designed dusting fabric that has a magnetic charge, or a damp, oiled cloth, and a damp mop to pick up dust particles.
- Wash walls, ceilings and floors frequently and wipe moldings, light fixtures, shelves and the tops of windows and doors.
- Replace wallpaper that shows traces of mold.
- If severely allergic, avoid basement apartments and bedrooms.
- Strip carpeting out of bedrooms.
- Never put carpeting in perennially damp areas.
- Make basements carpet-free if possible. (A carpet over a cement basement floor is one of the best places to grow a healthy mold or mite colony.)
- As vacuuming doesn't remove mites (which cling to fibers with their tiny feet), try killing them with an acaricide such as benzyl benzoate first, before vacuuming. Consider treating carpets with tannic acid to reduce cat allergens. (Some experts promote these measures; others consider them expensive and of temporary benefit only.)

Places where molds tend to lurk

Outdoors

- freshly mown grass
- piles of leaves
- composters and compost heaps
- poorly drained areas
- woodpiles
- haystacks and grain bins
- garbage cans
- camping equipment – sleeping bags, tents, boat cushions
- lawnmowers
- golf bags
- cars – under floor mats, in the air-conditioning system

Indoors:

- hotels and motels, recently opened cottages
- unfinished basements
- crawl spaces and attics
- utility rooms
- shower stalls and soap dishes
- cracks between bathroom tiles
- shower curtains
- magazines left in the bathroom
- refrigerator coils or drip trays
- window moldings
- aquariums
- soil around potted plants
- air-conditioners, dehumidifiers, humidifiers and vaporizers
- furnace filters
- damp closets
- damp shoes and boots
- surfaces soiled by children or pets
- foods and food cupboards – especially dried fruit, vegetables, old bread, aged cheese, pickled foods, beer, wine, vinegar and soy sauce

- Make the bedroom a pet-free zone, or at least make sure pets stay off beds.
- Vacuum and dust the home, car and office frequently, using a vacuum with HEPA filtration.
- Keep room humidity below 30 percent with a dehumidifier or air-conditioning unit.
- Use an exhaust fan in the bathroom to cut moisture and prevent buildup of molds.

- Wash kitchen and bathroom surfaces with mold-killing bleach or cleaner at least once monthly.
- Leave doors between rooms open to maximize air flow.
- Change or clean filters on the cooling and heating systems about once a month.
- Clean dehumidifiers weekly.
- Keep allergic people out of the room while cleaning.
- Keep external areas near the house dry and free of organic wastes, which are a prime breeding ground for molds.
- Use a clothes dryer rather than an outdoor clothesline so clothes don't collect pollen.
- Protect mattresses and pillows with special vinyl or plastic covers, zipped and taped shut. Choose furniture made of wood, metal, leather or plastic. Eliminate dust-catching stuffed furniture. Keep floors bare or use small, easily washable, synthetic throw rugs. Make sure any carpets and underpads are made of synthetic material, with short pile – never shag.
- Use pillows filled with hypoallergenic material, synthetic or foam – avoid feathers and kapok.
- Use comforters and blankets made with hypoallergenic material, washable cotton or synthetics, instead of wool or natural down.
- Wash blankets and bedspreads weekly, and sheets and pillowcases more often, if possible. Wash bedding in very hot water (130°F, or 55°C). Cool water does not kill dust mites.
- Choose mattresses made of synthetic material.
- Vacuum mattresses each time sheets are changed.
- Avoid dust-collecting venetian blinds and shutters, and dust-catchers such as hangings, pennants, chalkboards and open shelving.
- Choose synthetic fibers for curtains or use washable blinds. Use curtains that are short, light, smooth and easily washable.

- Store out-of-season clothing and supplies in boxes or tightly zippered garment bags.
- Treat carpets and upholstered furniture with an anti-allergen dust spray to neutralize dust-mite allergens, pet dander and pollens.
- Arrange furniture so it can be easily dusted.
- Ventilate kitchens and bathrooms well; wash under sinks and behind toilets and clean frequently with chlorine bleach (including tiles and grout).
- Try insecticides to kill cockroaches.
- Fix leaky plumbing and seal cracks where water can leak in, as mold forms where there is dampness.

EIGHT

Allergies in Children

Allergy is a leading cause of ill health in children and, although rarely life-threatening, childhood allergies can be severe. About 10 to 15 percent of children in North America suffer from one or more allergies, most commonly atopic dermatitis (eczema) and food allergies. Eczema affects about 15 percent of children under one year old and 5 percent of schoolchildren. And about 3 percent of North American children have food allergies, especially to cow's milk, eggs, soy, wheat, fish and increasingly peanuts. The numbers are higher in children from allergic families, among whom 7 percent have an identified cow's milk allergy. Pollen allergies tend to appear later in childhood, around age eight to ten. Some studies suggest that the month of birth makes a difference to the type and extent of childhood allergies. Exposure to pollens within the first few months of birth may increase the risk of hay fever. In Scandinavian studies, children born from February to April were more likely to be allergic to birch pollen, and those delivered from April to May were more often allergic to grass pollens than those born in winter months. Presumably, these children were sensitized to pollens soon after birth.

Parents are encouraged to learn how to recognize allergic conditions, and how to protect their children from allergies. Infants are especially prone to food allergies because their immature immune and digestive systems are not yet fully able to handle "foreign" food proteins. Allergy-prone parents can try to prevent or postpone allergies in their offspring by breast-feeding for as long as possible (six to nine months), avoiding allergenic foods while nursing and delaying the introduction of solids, particularly known allergy-provokers such as cow's milk, eggs, peanuts and seafood. Parents should inform school authorities if their child has a serious allergy, so that appropriate precautions can be taken.

Key Childhood Allergies

- *Atopic dermatitis* (eczema) is far more frequent in infants and young children than in adults. Children prone to atopic dermatitis almost always have their first attack in infancy. An estimated 10 to 15 percent of children aged four months to one year, and 5 percent of schoolchildren, have eczema, about one-third coming from allergy-prone families, but 75 percent outgrow it by the time they are teenagers. (See also Chapter Twelve.)
- *Food allergies* – in particular to cow's milk and eggs – are more common in infants and children than in adults. In North America and Europe about 2 to 3 percent of children under age three (up to 7 percent in allergy-prone families) are suspected of having an IgE-mediated cow's milk allergy.
- *Urticaria* (hives) occurs in roughly 20 percent of children, not just from allergies but often from viral infections, as a reaction to medications and from other causes.
- *Asthma* affects an estimated 10 percent of pre-adolescent children.

- *Insect-sting allergy* – severe, possibly life-threatening reactions to insect stings – affects less than 1 percent of children (compared to 3 percent of adults). Insect-sting deaths are rare in children. Even children who have had a severe anaphylactic insect-sting reaction may not react on being stung again. But experts stress that, even though an insect sting sensitivity may seem to have faded or been outgrown, this *cannot be relied upon*, and precautions must *always* be taken if the child is stung again, as anaphylaxis could recur.
- *Seasonal hay fever and perennial (year-round) rhinitis* are less common in infants than in older children. Allergies to pollens, dust, animal dander and other inhalants increase as children get older, affecting as many as 10 to 20 percent of teens and adults.
- *Drug allergies* are uncommon in children, as they are exposed to fewer drugs, although allergy-like (but not IgE-mediated) reactions to antibiotics are common. Parents frequently misattribute miscellaneous rashes to a drug allergy.
- *Contact dermatitis* is rare in children, although young children can be sensitized to topical products such as skin creams or perfumed soaps.

Recognizing Allergies in Children

Many of the signs and symptoms of allergy in children are easily confused with those due to other ailments, so that the condition is hard to diagnose. For example, vomiting and diarrhea may signal a food allergy, but could equally well be a symptom of gastroenteritis, bacterial food poisoning, influenza or a food intolerance. A 1992 study reported in *The New England Journal of Medicine* looked at life-threatening anaphylactic reactions in American children and found that, of six fatal cases of food-induced anaphylaxis, four occurred at school and went unrecognized, or were not treated with an

Common alerting signs of allergy in children

- *immediate vomiting* after eating a certain food or being stung (perhaps along with hives and face swelling);
- *hives on the face, arms, legs or body* – a frequent sign of childhood allergy but often due to a viral infection, or a drug reaction. Hives may break out immediately after the child takes a food or drug to which he or she has been sensitized;
- *spring and summertime sniffing, sneezing, itchy nose and red eyes* – resembling a drawn-out cold, but perhaps due to seasonal allergic rhinitis (hay fever);
- *a characteristic "allergic salute"* – the palm of the hand rubbed upwards against the tip of the nose to relieve itching – typical of children with hay fever;
- *a grimace or facial twitch;*
- *"allergic shiners"* (dark circles around or under the eyes) and a perpetually tired look due to hay fever or year-round allergic rhinitis – not to be confused with bluish patches under and above the eyes demarcated by a red line, which signals an eye condition called "orbital cellulitis" which requires immediate medical attention;
- *mouth-breathing and loud snoring,* often caused by nasal stuffiness or by enlarged adenoids;
- *wheezing* – a common sign of asthma, which may be allergy-provoked in older children but is more likely from a viral infection in infants. The definition of "wheezing" is hazy but the word generally refers to a whistling sound on breathing out;
- *atopic dermatitis, or infantile eczema* – an itchy, dry and scaling, or weepy, oozy rash on the cheeks, chin, even the outer arms and legs, or on any part of a child's body except the diaper area (which is usually moist and spared from scaly eczema). In older children the eczematous rash is drier and tends to occur in the creases behind the knees and in the elbows, and in the neck. Eczema is not always allergy-induced;
- *angioedema, or swelling of the skin's deeper layers,* especially of the mouth, lips, throat and vocal cords; this can be life-threatening and needs immediate medical attention.

epinephrine injection in time. Schools must be aware of students who have a potentially life-threatening allergic reaction; school personnel must know how to recognize the signs and symptoms, and what to do.

Children Tend to Outgrow Early Allergies

Many children, even those with infant allergies, outgrow their allergies as they get older – especially eczema and certain food allergies. In one 1987 U.S. study, 8 percent of children had adverse reactions to various foods, and an estimated 3 percent of these reactions were proven to be allergies. Overwhelmingly, the infants outgrew early food allergies, and by the time they were three years old 85 percent no longer reacted to the offending food triggers. As the child's immune system matures, it becomes more resistant to allergy-provoking proteins, and skin tests will reveal which have been outgrown and which persist.

In one frequently cited Colorado study, 80 percent of children's food allergies were gone by the age of three, but many of the children later developed other allergies such as hay fever, asthma or different food allergies. An early cow's milk allergy may vanish around age two only to be replaced later by an airborne allergy or asthma.

As discussed in Chapter One, the changing pattern of childhood allergies, with some being outgrown and others surfacing, is known as the "allergic march." Depending on the severity of their symptoms, children often outgrow allergies to wheat, eggs, milk and soy, but they are less likely to outgrow peanut, nut or shellfish allergies. Food allergies that start after age three are less likely to vanish or fade with increasing age. Unfortunately there is no test to predict whether a particular child will develop or outgrow an allergy. As the child gets older, challenge tests will help to determine whether he or she can eat previously forbidden items.

How Children Get Sensitized

Since a baby can make IgE antibodies even before birth, in theory the baby could become sensitized to foods eaten by the mother during pregnancy. Some experts believe that such *in utero* sensitization is one possible reason for early infant allergies, although only isolated instances of pre-birth sensitization have been verified. In general, allergists consider fetal sensitization possible but "rare, at most," in the words of one pediatric allergist. In his view, "restricting maternal diets during the third trimester (last third) of pregnancy will not prevent most infant allergies, so it seems inappropriate and futile to limit an expectant woman's diet in the hope of forestalling her child's possible allergy." Not only may an allergen-restricted diet during pregnancy fail to prevent infant allergy, but the restriction may jeopardize the mother's (and the developing baby's) nutritional wellbeing.

Scientists are searching for better ways to identify children at risk of developing allergies, not only through family history but also by predictive tests such as measurement of antibody levels in cord blood before birth, and newborn allergy tests – so far with little success. Initial enthusiasm for measuring cord-blood levels of IgE in late pregnancy has been dampened by recent studies showing it to be a poor allergy predictor. Measuring IgE antibody levels in the blood of newborns may more accurately show which children are likely to develop allergies. In some studies, 75 percent of infants under a year old who had high blood IgE levels later developed one or more allergies.

Low-allergen Diets for Breastfeeding Mothers

While allergic sensitization during fetal life is considered rare, sensitization during breastfeeding, through food consumed by the mother, is common and is being increasingly identified. Many allergists recommend that breastfeeding mothers avoid allergenic foods, in particular cow's milk, eggs, peanuts, nuts, soy, fish, shellfish and perhaps beef. Several studies suggest that infant eczema is less likely to occur if the mother takes these precautions. In one study, half of 97 mothers who breastfed their babies for six months

The debate over breastfeeding and allergies

Prolonged breastfeeding – for six or more months – may reduce or delay the appearance of allergies such as infant eczema (atopic dermatitis) in the first three years of life. Studies find that premature babies fed banked human breastmilk rather than cow's milk formula have lower blood histamine levels and less risk of developing allergic diseases. The protective effects of breastmilk may stem partly from its various antibodies, which may inhibit IgE production. However, opinions are divided about the value of prolonged breastfeeding as an allergy-preventing strategy. Although it undoubtedly confers many nutritional benefits, and breastmilk is the optimal baby food for the first six months after birth, studies of the efficacy of breastfeeding in preventing or delaying allergies have had mixed results. Some studies were poorly designed – not well controlled ("randomized") – so they may have given inaccurate results.

In general, allergists believe prolonged breastfeeding postpones rather than prevents the development of allergies. Nonetheless, it can sharply reduce the risk of infant eczema, a condition distressing to both baby and parents. Studies show that infants from allergy-prone families fed only breastmilk for the first six months after birth had far less eczema than those started on cow's milk and solids at the age of three to four months. (See also Chapter Twelve.)

ate no milk, eggs, soy, fish or peanuts during lactation, while the other half ate whatever they liked. The incidence of infant eczema in the babies of mothers with restricted diets was about half that in the babies of mothers who ate as they pleased.

However, breastfeeding mothers who adopt hypoallergenic diets should seek professional dietary advice to make sure they don't shortchange themselves (or their babies) of essential nutrients. They must also realize that, while nutritional restriction may postpone the appearance of allergies, and reduce the incidence of infant allergies, it's unlikely to prevent allergies altogether. Studies find that, by age seven, even the children of mothers who restricted their diets while breastfeeding do not stay allergy-free. Most have only a temporary reprieve – albeit a welcome one – from allergic disorders.

Delaying the Introduction of Solid Foods May Also Help

Studies show that, besides breastfeeding for at least six months, not giving supplemental solid foods or fresh cow's milk during this time can also help to prevent or delay the appearance of allergic disorders in children. Allergy-prone infants who drink cow's milk formula in the first few months after birth often develop a cow's milk allergy. Many allergists suggest taking great care in weaning children at risk of allergies from breast-milk, and giving no allergenic foods until the child's first birth-day. That may mean no cow's milk, eggs, citrus fruits or wheat for the first year. Some allergists suggest excluding egg, peanuts, and fish and other seafood until the child is three years of age. Peanut products might even be taboo until a child reaches the age of five.

Despite all possible preventive efforts, some children have an allergic reaction to milk, eggs, peanut butter or other foods the very first time they're fed these items. If the children were not sensitized through the mother's breastmilk they may have been inadvertently exposed to traces of foodstuffs they licked or tasted.

Dealing with Cow's Milk Allergy in Young Children

Cow's milk allergy affects 1 to 3 percent of North American children under three years old, with symptoms – such as vom-iting, diarrhea, gastrointestinal distress, respiratory difficulty and hives – usually appearing within an hour of ingesting cow's milk proteins. The child may be sensitive to specific milk pro-teins such as whey and casein. The milk sensitivity often wanes around 18 months of age, as the immune system and gastric tract mature. (Less than 1 percent of North American adults are allergic to cow's milk.)

Parental smoking may increase allergy risks

The children of smoking parents not only are at increased risk of wheezing, respiratory problems and middle-ear infections, but may also have greater risks of developing early allergies (such as asthma) and a higher chance of getting pollen and food allergies. Children exposed to second-hand tobacco smoke in the home tend to have reduced growth rates, impaired lung function, more atopic dermatitis and an earlier onset of allergic rhinitis. Many studies have shown above-average IgE levels in the children of tobacco smokers. The evidence suggests increased allergic sensitization in children with early exposure to tobacco smoke – strong incentive for parents to stop smoking!

The best substitute for cow's milk when a baby is being weaned from the breast is much debated. In the past, infants allergic to cow's milk were often switched to soy formula; however, recent studies find that some infants allergic to cow's milk also develop a soy allergy. Nonetheless, soy remains a cheap and commonly used cow's milk substitute. Among the other formula substitutes available are *casein hydrolysates*: hypoallergenic formulas made by heat-treating cow's milk to break down its bovine proteins into smaller, less allergy-provoking fractions. Casein hydrolysate formulas have been available for many years and may be well tolerated by infants allergic to cow's milk. Newer, reportedly better-tasting and less expensive products now on the market include *whey hydrolysates*. However, these newer products may be somewhat less well tolerated than the older ones.

When switching from breastmilk to formula, parents can now choose from a wide selection of non-allergenic formulas, with the advice of their pediatrician or other caregivers. Feeding allergy-prone infants with hypoallergenic formula rather than cow's milk may delay the onset of eczema and gastric food allergy. However, allergists stress that for children allergic to cow's milk, the substitute may not be entirely risk-free; "hypoallergenic" does *not* mean "nonallergenic." On rare occasions, severe reactions to hypoallergenic formulas have been documented in infants with cow's milk allergy.

Choosing the Right Baby Formula

A quick inspection of today's pharmacies will reveal a confusing diversity of commercially prepared infant formulas. The three main categories are classified according to their protein sources. They contain either cow's milk protein, hydrolyzed (predigested) milk protein or soy protein. Numerous variations of these three types have been specially designed for specific infant-feeding problems, such as cow's milk allergy. Among the much-debated points about baby formula are its optimal iron and fatty acid content, when to replace regular cow's milk formula with alternative forms, how long to continue formula-feeding and when to introduce fresh cow's milk.

The alternatives to cow's milk formulas include:

- *lactose-free formulas,* useful for infants who are "lactose-intolerant" – intolerant to the lactose (sugar) in cow's milk. This condition is shown by symptoms such as excessive gas, abdominal bloating and diarrhea. Since the symptoms of lactose intolerance can mimic those of a milk allergy, tests may be done to distinguish the two. With a milk-protein allergy, a baby may develop eczema, hives, flushing, swollen lips and other symptoms. For a lactose-intolerant baby with no signs of milk-protein allergy, a lactose-free, milk-protein formula will serve. Lactose-free formulas include *soy-protein* and *hydrolyzed casein* formulas. For a baby who is milk-allergic as well as lactose-intolerant, special hydrolysate formula may be advised.

Key types of formula

Standard	Cow's-milk-based. May contain lactose.
Iron-fortified	Cow's-milk-based. May contain lactose.
Lactose-free	Cow's-milk-based but lactose-free, for infants with feeding problems due to lactose intolerance.
Soy	Milk-free, soy-based formula, useful for infants with a milk protein allergy. Lactose-free. May contain sucrose or be sucrose-free. Should be used with physician advice.
Hypoallergenic or *hydrolyzed*	A hypoallergenic formula specially designed for infants with colic, or those who cannot tolerate milk-based or soy-protein-based formulas. Lactose-free.

- *soy-protein formulas,* the principal alternative to cow's milk formula for milk-allergic babies, but not suitable for premature infants. Soy formulas are lactose-free so they are also good for infants with lactose intolerance, milk allergy and galactosemia (an inherited inability to metabolize the milk sugar *galactose*). The carbohydrates used in most soy formulas are sucrose and corn syrup, easily digestible by infants. But soy formula may not be the right choice for infants allergic to milk protein because of the possibility of cross-reactivity – an allergic reaction to proteins in both soy and cow's milk. A soy-protein allergy may be suspected if the infant's symptoms (such as hives, diarrhea and wheezing) are not relieved within a few days of switching from cow's milk to soy formula.
- *hydrolyzed-protein formulas,* suitable for babies with a cow's milk-protein allergy and as "specialty" formulas for severe feeding problems and nutritional disorders. Although hydrolyzed-protein formulas are made from

cow's milk, the milk protein is first broken into its component amino acids – basically "predigested" – decreasing the likelihood of allergic reactions. However, these formulas are expensive and many physicians suggest trying other forms first.

Be Wary of Elimination Diets

Once a childhood food allergy is diagnosed, the best treatment is to eliminate the offending food from the diet. But it's wise to seek the advice of a trained nutritionist or pediatrician before putting your child on an elimination diet. While such a diet can prevent severe symptoms, the replacement diet must be nutritionally sound. Unusual or very restricted diets can deprive young children of vital nutrients and lead to malnutrition. Usually, only one or two foods need be avoided; only rarely is it necessary to eliminate more. One British case illustrates the hazards of an unduly restrictive anti-allergy diet. A four-year-old was taken to an alternative therapist who diagnosed "multiple food sensitivity" and prescribed a "hypoallergenic diet" excluding dairy products, with no eggs, no chocolate, no sugar, fish, beef, lamb or pork. After several months on the diet, the child's growth became stunted. A pediatrician who examined the child diagnosed hypothyroidism due to a lack of dietary iodine. Only very rarely are broad exclusion diets advised for children.

Behavior Problems in Allergy-prone Children

Although psychological and emotional problems do not cause atopic dermatitis or other allergies, allergic disorders can lead to psychological difficulties, especially in children. In one 1992 study, 25 percent of children with severe asthma had emotional problems. This confirmed the findings of a 1991 survey showing that half the asthmatic children investigated found

> ## Testing whether a food allergy has faded
>
> To determine whether a child has outgrown a non-life-threatening allergy, physicians may try a "controlled challenge test," in which a small amount of the food in question is placed on the child's lips. If there is no reaction, the amount is slowly increased. If the child can eat a normal serving without reacting, "tolerance" has developed to that particular food, and it can thereafter be eaten normally. Food challenge tests may be done after the age of one year, and can be repeated every six months to a year. But challenge tests – especially food challenge tests – require great care; they should only be done by a physician in a medical office, with emergency equipment on hand in case of severe reactions.

the disorder a major hindrance in their home and school lives. Children with severe allergies may be not only distressed by the discomfort of a persistently itchy skin or irrepressible sneezing, but also ashamed of a rash, or disabled by asthmatic wheezing, and plagued by embarrassment. An allergic disorder may keep them from taking part in the usual sports and other activities. Parents or teachers who suspect that a child is emotionally stressed, or has problems coping with an allergic disorder, should seek the advice of a certified allergist or a family physician and obtain suitable counseling.

Signs of Emotional Problems Due to Allergies
- persistent anxiety
- difficulties with schoolwork
- sleeping problems
- emotional withdrawal, apathy
- depression
- changes in a child's behavior – e.g., disobedience or "acting out" (venting frustration through hostility)
- symptoms worsening despite good medical care

Colic and allergy

Many a parent dreads "colic" – persistent, inconsolable crying for no apparent reason. Classic colic starts up when a baby is about two weeks old and may mean several hours of crying daily . Disruptive, stressful, frustrating and annoying, severe colic can drive parents to distraction in their efforts to quiet the baby. (Peak sounds of infant screams during a colic attack have registered up to 117 decibels, just below the sound of a jackhammer.)

Colic can stem from various causes, including poor feeding habits such as swallowing too much air while feeding, or from an allergy or intolerance to cow's milk, soy or other formula. Although many parents believe colic is due to a milk allergy or "something wrong with the milk," very rarely is infant colic related to the milk. Sometimes severe colic improves when a baby is taken off cow's milk formula and put onto a hypoallergenic brand, but in many cases changing the formula fails to ease the problem. It's not easy to predict which babies will get better with a change of formula. One pediatrician suggests that, for infants with very severe daily crying, changing from cow's milk or soy formula to a hypoallergenic type for a few days can demonstrate whether the crying stops and the infant improves, and whether a long-term switch might be worthwhile. Although colic is not IgE-mediated, a few British studies suggest that it may occasionally be a sign of allergy; however, this remains to be confirmed.

Allergies Are Unpredictable

Sophie, Susie and Cass were all from strongly allergy-prone families and had partners with allergies. When they became pregnant, all three women consulted their physicians, who advised them that, based on their family histories, the chance of their infants developing allergies was about 70 percent. Because they were identified as "high risk," these women were advised to breastfeed their infants for at least six months and, while nursing, to eliminate from their diets certain allergy-provoking foods, such as milk, eggs, seafood and peanuts, not to smoke and not to be exposed to smoke at home. Sophie didn't take the advice. She found breastfeeding too time-consuming, particularly as she needed to return to work, so she put her baby on formula at three months of age. The child developed a serious cow's milk allergy and, feeling guilty, Sophie blamed herself. Susie, in contrast, followed the allergist's advice scrupulously. She breastfed her child for six months, adding solid food only after that, and she herself maintained a rigorous diet and asked her husband not to smoke. Nevertheless, Susie's child developed eczema. Cass, on the other hand, took none of the advice and ate what she liked, switching her infant from breastmilk to cow's milk formula after two months. Yet her child is still allergy-free at eight years old. The moral of the story: allergies are unpredictable. You have to weigh the risks and benefits and make a personal choice, realizing that preventive strategies are worth following but not foolproof, and offer no absolute guarantee of preventing or even postponing childhood allergies.

Treating Childhood Allergy

Antihistamines and decongestants used for adult allergies can also be used in children, although in lower doses. (Dosing recommendations are listed on the package. Note that the "half life" of the drug may be longer in children; they may need to wait longer between doses.)

- *Antihistamines.* Older forms such as chlorpheniramine can cause drowsiness, so the newer nonsedating forms may be preferable. The choice should be discussed with the child's physician.
- *Decongestants* such as pseudoephedrine or phenylpropanolamine (used alone or alongside antihistamines) are considered safe for healthy children, but should be used with caution in those with seizures, heart disease or high blood pressure.
- *Cromolyn* is a very safe drug with few side-effects, although nasal irritation can be a problem for some young children.

- *Inhaled corticosteroids* are safe and effective medications, although very young children have trouble using sprays or metered-dose inhalers, and some don't tolerate nasal sprays well. School-age children have less trouble.
- *Corticosteroid creams and ointments* for skin rashes, frequently prescribed for infants and children, are safe and effective provided low-potency products are used – with caution in young children, as the drug can be absorbed through the skin into the bloodstream.
- *Immunotherapy (allergy injections)* is not recommended for children under five as the procedure could cause serious reactions in young children. However, for older children immunotherapy against specific pollens, insect venoms, cats or mites can work well.

Strategies That May Reduce Allergies in At-Risk Children

- *Obtain expert advice* to determine the risk for the child, and work out an allergy-reducing strategy.
- *Ban smoking* in the home and avoid exposure to second-hand tobacco smoke.
- *Decrease exposure to dust and molds* as much as possible.

Diet Tips

- *Breastfeed for six to nine months if possible.*
- *While breastfeeding, eat a generally non-allergenic diet,* avoiding eggs, milk, shellfish and peanuts, but seek nutritional advice about replacing these nutrient-rich foods.
- *Delay introducing solid foods for six months if possible,* and add less allergenic foods first. Give no eggs until 18 months of age, and no peanut products until the child is at least three years old.
- *Introduce new foods one at a time,* observing the child's

reaction and looking for possible allergy symptoms (ask the pediatrician what to look for).

Making the Child's Bedroom Dust-Free

- *Replace the stuffing* of a much-loved toy by cutting it open along a seam, emptying it before washing and refilling with nylon stockings or synthetic material such as polyester fiberfill.
- *Choose toys* that are easily washable – plastic, metal or wooden – and keep them in an enclosed box, drawer or cabinet.
- *Move as much as possible* of the furniture, carpets, clothes, toys and books out of the bedroom – it should contain no carpets, rugs, mats, stored blankets, books, stuffed toys or clutter. "One toy, preferably a washable one, and one book may be taken to bed at night," suggests one expert.
- *Seal the hot air vent* with duct tape. Heat the room with an electric baseboard radiator or hot water heater.
- *Install a bare* vinyl or hardwood floor.
- *Enclose mattress and box spring* in a zippered cover.
- *Limit bedding to synthetic fiber* or foam-chip pillows, a mattress pad, sheets, cotton thermal or synthetic fiber blankets and quilts. Launder these every two to four weeks in hot water (140°F or 60°C).
- *In bunk beds*, make sure an allergic child has the upper berth.
- *If there is a chest of drawers*, clean the drawers every few months.
- *Explain*, when the child is old enough, why animals cannot be allowed in the bedroom, or perhaps even in the house.
- *If humidification is necessary*, keep the relative humidity below 30 percent. Scrub the humidifier with soap and water every two weeks.

- *Try to have the child out of the house while vacuuming.*
  As living rooms are notoriously dusty, encourage the child
  to play in other areas, such as the kitchen or family room
  or, better still, out of doors.

If you find some of these measures impractical in your home,
at least encase the mattress and box spring in plastic and wash
the blankets and pillows regularly (see Chapter Seven).

Parents who are considering opting for an allergy-preventing
plan must consider the time and effort involved. For example,
eliminating allergy-causing items from the diet not only limits
nutrition but also requires more imagination in cooking and
additional preparation, and may cause problems when you
dine out. Hypoallergenic formulas are more expensive than
cow's milk, and some infants don't like them. Considering
such inconveniences and the lack of any proof that a hypoallergenic lifestyle can ultimately prevent allergies, some experts
feel it's inappropriate to foist overly rigorous rules on parents
or other caregivers.

Protecting Children with Severe Allergies

The Canadian Society of Allergy and Clinical Immunology
has issued new guidelines to help schools prevent and deal
with severe anaphylactic reactions through education, early
recognition and prompt treatment of potentially life-threatening reactions. A 1995 report from the society suggests that
schools develop a system for identifying children with life-
threatening allergies. Most fatalities occur away from home,
usually because epinephrine was not used, or not used soon
enough. All teachers must know about students who could
require epinephrine. U.S. guidelines are similar and the American Academy of Allergy, Asthma and Immunology is adopt-
ing the Canadian school guidelines.

Children prone to anaphylaxis must be properly identified and their allergy clearly stated (e.g., on a medical-alert bracelet). Identification sheets could include the child's name, photograph and specific allergy. (Information and identification sheets are available from the Anaphylaxis Project of the Canadian Allergy/Asthma Information Association and similar U.S. organizations.) Parents can sign a waiver allowing the school to use epinephrine when it's considered necessary. Every child given an auto-injector kit should label it with his or her name and keep it readily available. Because of the potential suddenness and severity of allergic shock, children cannot always administer the drug themselves; they may need help from a teacher or other caregiver. Epinephrine is needed *as soon as* a child develops any allergy symptoms, and the child must be taken to hospital immediately for monitoring.

Schools should have on hand first-aid kits that contain epinephrine auto-injectors in designated areas (e.g., lunch rooms, gymnasiums, schoolyards, swimming pools). The devices should be handy and accessible (*not* in locked cabinets) in case of need. In one study, children who died of anaphylaxis had been prescribed an EpiPen but did not have it on them when the anaphylactic reaction occurred, or delayed using it. Parents of children with life-threatening allergies must make sure their offspring carry the auto-injector with them *at all times*, and know how to use it.

Children can be allergic to many substances, but among the most lethal are foods, in particular fish, shellfish, peanuts and tree nuts (such as hazelnuts, walnuts, almonds and cashews). "It cannot be stressed enough," notes one emergency physician, "that minute amounts of these foods (often as hidden ingredients) can be life-threatening. Several children have had frightening anaphylactic episodes from residual peanut butter or bits of fish left on tables." The number of anaphylactic episodes in children is increasing, and so our need for awareness is growing too. Many people at risk of anaphylaxis have already had severe hives, swelling and respiratory distress after eating a food to which they're allergic. Many seriously food-allergic children also have asthma. However, studies show that children who die of anaphylaxis can have deceptively mild symptoms at first.

To make schools and daycare centers safer for allergic children, teachers, staff and parents must recognize the possible severity of allergic reactions to food and other allergens. It takes only traces – even the residue left on a knife used to spread peanut butter – to trigger a life-threatening reaction.

Helping Schools Handle Allergy Problems

While allergic disorders in primary-school children should be discussed with the school staff, some experts suggest extreme tact at the secondary level, as broadcasting an allergy problem could embarrass older children. With modern medications, most allergies can be managed in a way that permits children to live a normal life. Parents should tell the school about the severity of a child's allergy but not overdramatize it, explaining the possibility of anaphylactic shock and the suggested precautions. Teachers who are aware of a potential health problem can be prepared for and understand a child's behavior, which might otherwise seem to be "attention seeking."

Given careful management, children with allergies can go to camp, join sports teams, play tennis, swim and sleep over at a friend's house. If they are dealt with honestly and allowed to participate fully in school activities, they develop self-confidence and need not feel diminished by their allergies. On the other hand, they should not be unduly pampered or made to feel special, as they could become manipulative and demanding, and might even refuse to take medication in order to attract

---

Preventive strategies for children with food allergies

Children with food allergies should be taught to:

- avoid sharing food, and not trade utensils or food containers;
- wash their hands before and after eating;
- if known to be at risk, carry an auto-injector kit (and know how to use it), and wear a medical-alert bracelet or necklace stating that ana-phylaxis is possible;
- eat home-prepared lunches and snacks whenever possible;
- learn to read ingredient lists for themselves;
- ask about all ingredients in meals prepared elsewhere before ordering or eating them. Some restaurants provide ingredient lists and have someone on hand to answer questions. (See Chapter Ten for more tips.)

---

attention. Allergic kids should receive the same discipline as their siblings. The less they are made to feel "different," the better they can cope and develop their capacities.

Helping Allergy-prone Adolescents Cope

Children are best encouraged to take increasing responsibility for managing their disease as they reach adolescence, to help them develop self-confidence and life skills. Most high school students should be ready, willing and able to take responsibility for their health problems, just as they look after their personal hygiene. By the teen years there should be little need for parents to interfere at school. In fact, if parents intervene and discuss an adolescent's allergy too intensely with school staff, it could worsen matters by:

- labeling the parent "overprotective," destroying credibility;
- alienating a child who is trying to minimize his or her differences from peers.

Adolescents with allergies easily become discouraged. They want to get on with their lives, without the hassle of medication and being constantly on alert. Striving for autonomy and acceptance, teens are notorious risk-takers, and they may test the limits by neglecting to take allergy medication – or smoking, perhaps worsening the symptoms. There is often a strong drive to underestimate or even dismiss a serious or potentially lethal condition. Denial and complacency can have serious, even life-threatening consequences for those at risk of anaphylaxis or severe asthma. By neglecting their limitations, teens increase their risk of a severe episode, and when they need help there may be no one around who recognizes the danger or knows what to do about it. "Any parent or caregiver who has failed to openly discuss allergy control with the kids is asking for trouble," notes one allergist. "Still, parents are best advised not to be overprotective. If they try to shield adolescents from all risks, they shield them from the task of becoming independent, taking responsibility and maturing."

New treatment methods make allergy management easier than in the past. For example, various inhalers have significantly improved asthma and rhinitis treatment. Peak flow meters help give early-warning signs of worsening asthma, and epinephrine kits provide instant help for insect stings or a life-threatening food or drug allergy, and may even save a life. The best way to prevent minor allergic problems from becoming major ones is to enhance communication – between children and their friends, and with parents, teachers, counselors, babysitters, the family physician and other caregivers.

NINE

Understanding Asthma

A sthma – the name means "gasping for breath" – is a disorder in which inflammatory changes, muscle spasm and excess mucus secretion obstruct the breathing tubes, or airways, hindering the movement of air in and out of the lungs. A classic asthma attack surfaces with persistent coughing, wheezing, chest tightness and excess phlegm (mucus). It's an ancient disease, mentioned as far back as 1550 B.C.; Egyptian papyri suggest herbs and crocodile or camel excreta as remedies. In the third millennium B.C., Chinese medical men treated asthma with extracts of the *ma huang* plant, from which the modern decongestant drug ephedrine was later extracted. It was first called a breathing disorder by the ancient Greek physician Hippocrates, and the first book on asthma, written at the end of the 17th century, described its triggers – such as respiratory infections, exercise, irritants, stress and even laughter – noting its tendency to worsen at night and in the dawn hours.

Asthma is the commonest chronic childhood respiratory disease in North America. While some people suffer attacks only in childhood, the disease often recurs during adulthood. A few people first develop asthma as adults; some likely had undiagnosed childhood asthma. Over a million Canadians and 14 to 15 million Americans suffer from asthma. In the U.S., 1.8 million seek emergency care each year for an acute attack, with 4,000 to 5,000 asthma deaths annually (and 400 to 500 in Canada), many of them in persons under 25 years old.

Since 1980, the annual hospitalization rate for asthma in North America has increased by 28 percent, and the number of asthma deaths among young people has more than doubled; somewhat more boys than girls are affected. Figures are comparable in many other industrialized nations. There is growing concern about the incidence and severity of asthma, and the fact that, as one expert from the International Asthma Council puts it, "asthma is one of the few treatable diseases with a climbing death rate, especially among children and young adults." Fortunately, the rate is now leveling off.

Asthma specialists blame the heavy toll of asthma partly on neglect in "getting the message out" – failure to teach people about asthma and its potential severity, and failure on the part of medical caregivers to put into effect modern asthma-management strategies. "Failure to implement the new treatment approaches leads to many needless deaths each year," says one U.S. respirologist.

The experts call for better communication with patients, families, physicians, and other caregivers about the disease, more emphasis on treating asthma as an inflammatory condition (see below), and the development of a personal "action plan" for each sufferer to implement in case of worsening symptoms. People with asthma need to understand the disease, be able to monitor its severity and take prompt action if and when needed. Asthma *can* be controlled by proper management.

What Is Asthma?

Asthma is a sometimes reversible obstructive lung disease in which the airways (breathing tubes) are overly sensitive, or "twitchy." A group of Canadian experts who developed a set of 1996 recommendations for asthma management define the disease as "a disorder of the airways characterized by paroxysmal or persistent symptoms (shortness of breath, wheeze and coughing), with diminished air flow and airway 'hyperresponsiveness' [overreaction] in response to various stimuli."

In other words, asthma is a lung problem that comes and goes, in which the airways become inflamed, leading to diminished air flow and troubled breathing. The inflamed airways are swollen and congested, and respond in an exaggerated manner to common irritants, allergens and other triggers. They may also contract – develop *bronchospasm* – narrowing further, making it hard to breathe out. The familiar whistling or wheezing sound occurs with the effort of exhaling through the obstructed, mucus-clogged airways. But not all people with asthma wheeze. In many cases, the chief sign is a persistent cough, especially at night and first thing in the morning.

Decades ago, physicians had already noticed that the lungs of people who died of asthma were markedly inflamed. Recent bronchoscope studies looking at lung washings (samples) find signs of inflammation – such as excess eosinophils (white blood cells) – in even mildly asthmatic people. Inflammation is now considered the underlying problem in asthma, but several processes contribute to the breathing problem.

The airway's mucosal lining becomes inflamed in response to some trigger or irritant, with release of mediators (such as histamine, leukotrienes and platelet-activating factor), producing swelling and congestion.

Excess eosinophils accumulate at the site, contributing to the inflammation.

Respiratory System

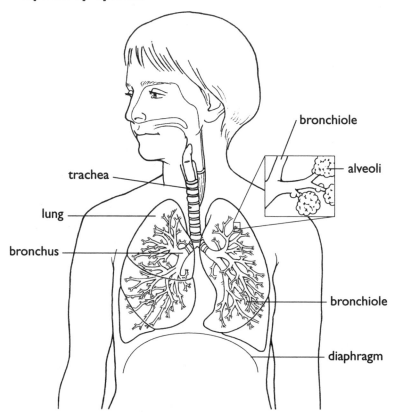

trachea

lung

bronchus

bronchiole

alveoli

bronchiole

diaphragm

How our lungs work

The lungs, the body's key respiratory organs, are constructed like two trees with innumerable branches. The windpipe, or *trachea*, divides into *bronchi*, and then into finer branches or *bronchioles*, ending in tiny air sacs or *alveoli*. Air entering through the bronchi passes into the alveoli, where the oxygen in the air is absorbed into the bloodstream to be circulated to the rest of the body. Waste materials such as carbon dioxide pass from the bloodstream into the alveoli and are exhaled through the bronchi. The alveoli provide a huge absorption area to ensure an efficient intake of oxygen and discharge of waste gases. The airways are lined by a delicate *mucosal* or lining membrane, with little *cilia* (hairs) that beat in unison to clear debris. Mucus is produced by cells and glands in the respiratory system, for lubrication and to trap debris.

Bronchospasm of the muscles encircling the bronchi narrows their *lumens* (passageways), further hindering the movement of air through the lungs.

An excess of sticky mucus produced by the irritated bronchial tissue adds to the obstruction.

Damaged cells shed by the inflamed lining tissues increase the blockage.

Together, the inflammation, narrowing, mucus and debris in the airways make breathing out difficult, producing the familiar wheeze as the asthmatic tries to force air out through clogged passages – rather like blowing through a straw.

"Inflammation is the underlying pathology [disease mechanism] in asthma," emphasizes one respirologist. "The airway narrowing and breathing difficulties are the end result. If the inflammation is left untreated, the bronchi become still more hyperreactive [twitchy], increasing the constriction. The more inflamed the breathing passages are, the greater the airway blockage is and the tougher it is to breathe." The extent of airway obstruction varies in different parts of the lung, but its overall impact is an accumulation of stale, unoxygenated air in the lungs, diminishing the body's oxygen supply.

Airways

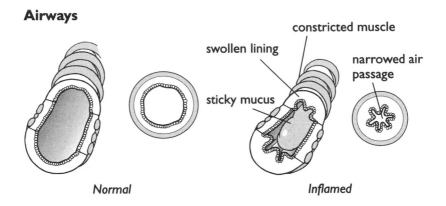

Normal

Inflamed

constricted muscle

swollen lining

narrowed air passage

sticky mucus

Oxygen shortage is the main danger of asthma

Since air passages are partially blocked in an asthma attack, the lungs cannot effectively push out the stale air with its load of waste carbon dioxide. The stale air trapped in the lungs prevents new oxygen-rich air from entering, leading to hypoxia or oxygen shortage throughout the body, and possibly acidosis (carbon dioxide buildup in the blood).

In its struggle to force the lungs to take in more oxygen, the brain drives the chest muscles to ever greater efforts, making asthmatics feel still more breathless. The use of auxiliary breathing muscles in the neck and abdomen and the indrawing of the muscles of the ribcage on inhaling can signal a severe attack. Serious oxygen depletion can be fatal if not given prompt medical attention.

How to Tell If You Have Asthma

Not every wheezer is asthmatic, and accurate diagnosis is essential for treatment. Telltale signs include a persistent cough (often worst at night and in the dawn hours), frequent and prolonged "chesty" colds, difficulty breathing, a wheezy or whistling sound, coughing up a lot of mucus (phlegm), perhaps the development of nasal polyps and frequent bouts of unusual pneumonia often unrelieved by antibiotics. Some people notice shortness of breath when they climb stairs, vacuum and so on. But since there may be no obvious physical signs, lung function (air-flow) tests are essential to gauge the extent of lung blockage.

The main diagnostic methods include

- medical history;
- physical examination – listening to the lungs with a stethoscope to detect airway obstruction. (The stethoscope amplifies the sound of air moving through the breathing tubes; if the bronchi are narrowed, the increased air-flow turbulence creates a higher-pitched sound. Fluid in the air sacs may produce a crackling noise);
- breathing tests to assess lung function;
- measurement of *peak expiratory flow rate (PEFR)* with a

peak flow meter, to assess the maximum speed at which air can be expelled from the lungs; this too demonstrates the extent of airway blockage;

* use of a *spirometer* – an instrument that measures the *forced expired volume (FEV)*, or the amount of air that can be blown out of the lungs, and other aspects of breathing out.

Breathing tests on asthmatics often reveal a reduced ability to force air out of the lungs. A repeat test, following a "puff" of bronchodilator (airway widener), may show increased air flow, helping to confirm the diagnosis. Since many asthmatics breathe normally when examined, testing with a mild bronchoconstrictor such as methacholine or histamine, which produces a controlled form of asthma, can often confirm a suspected case. Most asthmatic airways are remarkably sensitive to such inhaled substances and react with airway narrowing at relatively low doses. However, non-asthmatics also occasionally test positive.

Additional tests may include skin tests to identify allergic triggers, and chest X-rays.

Triggers That Can Set Off Attacks

Asthma may be triggered by intrinsic (internal) factors such as an inherited predisposition to twitchy breathing tubes, or by external (environmental) factors such as indoor air pollutants, pollens, animals, tobacco smoke or food or food additives. Some of these are allergens; others are non-allergic stimuli. In those prone to asthma, even exercise or cold air, or a viral infection such as a cold, influenza or bronchitis, often sets off an attack.

An estimated 40 to 60 percent of people with asthma are allergic to dust mites, pollens, food ingredients, molds, animal dander or other substances that provoke attacks. About 5 to

15 percent of asthmatics are allergic to ASA (called "aspirin" in the U.S.) and other nonsteroidal anti-inflammatory drugs (NSAIDs) – especially those who also have nasal polyps and sinusitis. But 40 to 50 percent of asthmatics have no known allergies, and asthma often has no identifiable trigger.

Tobacco smoke is a major asthma-provoker that can exacerbate airway inflammation and decrease the effectiveness of anti-asthma drugs. One expert in emergency medicine remarks that "about 10 to 20 percent of asthmatics are smokers who get into trouble through attacks aggravated by tobacco smoke." Secondhand smoke is also a known asthma trigger. Children who grow up in homes where people smoke are at increased risk of asthma, and tobacco smoke in the home can precipitate or worsen childhood attacks. Studies show that asthmatic children whose mothers smoke have twice as severe and frequent attacks as those living with non-smoking mothers.

Stress and emotions can increase the severity of an attack, but not cause one. Once an asthmatic attack begins, it may be aggravated by anxiety, frustration, fear, or even boisterous laughter – possibly a form of exercise-induced asthma.

Common Precipitating Triggers

- *respiratory tract infections* – e.g., viral head colds, acute bronchitis;
- *allergens* – aggravating about 50 percent of cases; at least half of all child asthmatics have known allergies, and suffer attacks when exposed to a specific allergen such as:
  - *dust mites*, in mattresses, bedding, stuffed toys, upholstered furniture, carpets, brooms, dusters or furnace filters
  - *pollens* from trees, grasses, weeds
  - *animal dander*, from rabbits, cats, dogs or hamsters, or the feathers of budgies and other birds

- *insect parts*, e.g., from cockroaches and certain flies
- *food triggers*, e.g., shellfish, peanuts, cow's milk
- *molds*, from trees, fallen leaves, home humidifiers, air-conditioners and ducts;
- *nocturnal factors* – exaggeration of the normal nighttime airway narrowing;
- *cigarette smoke*;
- *everyday pollutants and household irritants* such as car exhaust, paints, cleaning solvents, bleaches, detergents, furniture polish, deodorants;
- *exercise* – especially in winter and in cold, dry conditions; to reduce susceptibility cover the mouth and nose with a scarf when exercising in cold weather;
- *workplace or occupational irritants*;
- *weather changes* (e.g., fog, smog);
- *certain drugs* – especially ASA, other NSAIDs, beta blockers and some headache and glaucoma remedies;
- *certain food additives,* especially sulfite or metabisulfite preservatives used in wine, beer, juices, salad dressings and dried fruits.

Sensitivity to ASA and other NSAIDs

In sensitive asthmatics, ASA can trigger very severe attacks. Those sensitive to ASA usually react to all types of nonsteroidal anti-inflammatory drugs. Experts counsel such asthma sufferers to stay away from ASA products, other NSAIDs such as ibuprofen and certain analgesics. (ASA, or acetylsalicylic acid, is also known as "aspirin" in the U.S.) About 5 to 15 percent of asthmatics – especially those with the so-called allergic triad of asthma, nasal polyps and sinusitis – are extra-sensitive to such medications, perhaps because of some inherited biochemical change. Many over-the-counter medications contain ASA, which can trigger or aggravate asthma attacks by some mechanism that is, as yet, poorly understood. Alternatives such as acetaminophen are safer in such cases.

Workplace Triggers

Occupational exposure accounts for an estimated 4 percent of asthma cases. An early Greek reference to asthma noted that "mining dusts...stirred and beaten up...produce difficulty in breathing." Other classic examples of asthma-sensitizing chemicals are enzymes from the bacterium *Bacillus subtilis,* present in some detergents, and flour dust (a problem among bakers).

Today's prime culprits responsible for workplace asthma include

- wood dusts (especially cedar and hardwoods)
- accidental high-level exposure to some gases, including chlorine and sulfur dioxide
- soldering fumes
- latex
- isocyanates (used in certain paints, car seats and plastics)
- cereals, grains and their powders
- metals (platinum, chromium, nickel)

Workers with no known allergies may suddenly become wheezy on the job, even after years of working at the same place without breathing problems. One survey of employees at a platinum factory found that while some developed asthma after four months, others became asthmatic only after a decade of exposure. Latex is a new and increasing cause of occupational asthma.

Asthma Management Is Ideally a Joint Effort

In partnership with their physicians, asthmatics can learn to take charge and manage their condition. Once asthma has been diagnosed, the goal of treatment is to identify and (if possible) avoid the triggering agents, use medications to dampen symptoms and prevent flare-ups, and devise an action plan (preferably written down) for treating it and dealing with crisis situations early. Treatment usually works best when

Action plans: guidelines for self-management

An "action plan" is a simple, written set of instructions jointly created by physician and asthmatic, to be put into action any time the asthma worsens. Individually tailored to the person's symptoms, the action plan is based on peak flow readings and/or changes in symptoms (e.g., more coughing, chest tightness or wheezing). It aims to prevent severe attacks; the asthmatic must know how to use it. Usually simple enough to fit on a small index card, it includes precise instructions for the doses and types of medications to use, when to step up the frequency or size of doses, when to add or change medications and when to call the doctor or go to an emergency unit.

Generally, the action plan calls for increasing amounts of specific medication at signs of worsening or severe asthma – based on certain symptoms and a drop in self-measured peak flow rates. For instance, mild deterioration (perhaps a slight increase in breathlessness or disturbed sleep) may require more frequent or doubled doses of inhaled anti-inflammatory; if this strategy doesn't help in a day or two, other medication (perhaps a long-acting bronchodilator or a brief course of oral corticosteroids) may be added as step two, or the doctor may have to be consulted. The next step may be oral steroid tablets (kept at home and taken as instructed), and – if these don't help – a visit to the emergency unit. Signs of progressing severity may include a need for more bronchodilator puffs, greater breathlessness on exertion, nighttime coughing, peak expired flow rates below a certain level or failure of the changes in medication to bring relief. Use of a flow meter can help in gaining control as not all asthmatics know when they are getting sicker.

physician and patient work together to plan management of the disease, and to create the action plan.

Greater medical awareness of the key role of lung inflammation in asthma is gradually leading to better treatment and control. If you know you are sensitive to allergic or other asthma triggers, follow the environmental avoidance measures outlined elsewhere in this book, with special attention to mold and dust reduction – keeping your home well ventilated and at the right temperature and humidity levels. If you are sensitive to strong odors and industrial fumes, reduce your exposure to these irritants. All asthmatics should try to avoid tobacco smoke.

Pharmacotherapy

Asthma medications now allow good control for most asthmatics. Most anti-asthma drugs are inhaled forms that come in pocket-sized "puffers," convenient to carry and use. Inhaled drugs can be taken at lower doses than pills or syrups as they are absorbed directly into the lungs. New inhaler systems such as spacers and breath-activated "powder puffers" make anti-asthma drugs easier to use.

There are two main classes of anti-asthma medication.

- *Anti-inflammatory drugs* (both steroidal and nonsteroidal) – to mute or abolish the underlying inflammation – are taken regularly to keep symptoms at bay and stop attacks from surfacing. Anti-inflammatory medications are now increasingly recommended as "first-line" therapy, even as a preventive for mild asthmatics.
- *Bronchodilators*, which dilate (widen) narrowed airways, are used as needed for swift but temporary relief of breathing problems and for relieving flare-ups.

A combination of medications usually provides the best control, with the drug regime being carefully tailored to the individual's needs. For good management, and to help avoid severe attacks, it's essential to follow your physician's advice and take your medications as prescribed. If asthma interferes with your usual activities or keeps you awake at night, the treatment is inadequate and needs to be reviewed.

Those whose asthma remains troublesome despite adherence to "doctor's orders" should request a second opinion from a specialist, local asthma center or clinic. Simply tossing back more pills or taking more inhaler puffs without medical advice is *not* a sensible way to handle this disease.

Managing Asthma As an Inflammatory Disorder

The treatment of asthma has changed dramatically in recent years. While in the past the disease was thought to be mainly due to airway narrowing – calling for bronchodilator drugs as first-line therapy – today it's viewed as an *inflammatory condition* requiring primarily anti-inflammatory drugs. And while asthmatics formerly relied chiefly on routinely prescribed bronchodilator drugs, these drugs are now recommended only when symptoms worsen; anti-inflammatories are used regularly, sooner and more liberally than before, to control the underlying disorder. Both inhaled corticosteroids and nonsteroidal drugs such as nedocromil and cromolyn (which are considerably less effective) are used to suppress the inflammation; some nonsteroidal drugs also act as anti-allergy agents.

At a 1996 Canadian Asthma Consensus Conference, experts in allergy, lung disease and emergency medicine issued strong recommendations to "focus on reducing the inflammatory state through environmental control and early use of anti-inflammatory agents, rather than by symptomatic therapy [to widen airways] alone." So anti-inflammatory agents are becoming "state of the art" first-line asthma treatment, with bronchodilators as backup or "rescue" medications to be used "if and when needed," for the "shortest time possible, at the lowest possible dose."

Inhaled corticosteroids are considered the best agents for bringing and keeping asthma under control, and may also improve the long-term prognosis. Once the condition is stabilized, the lowest possible dose is used. However, many asthmatics are reluctant to take corticosteroid anti-inflammatories

> ## Inflammation is the problem
> "The main message to get across to asthmatics," stress the experts, "is that the problem in asthma is inflammation. That is what has to be treated. There is no point in using airway-widening drugs without paying attention to this primary cause, because the problems will only come back."

because they act more slowly and must be taken regularly.

Also, anxiety about possible ill effects has made both asthmatics and some of their caregivers hesitant about corticosteroids, even though they are among the most valuable asthma drugs available. Experts stress that although long-term corticosteroids taken by mouth may cause side-effects such as weight gain, fluid retention, hypertension, osteoporosis, diabetes and cataracts, inhaled corticosteroids act locally on the airway and little of the medication is absorbed into the bloodstream. In low to moderate doses, they cause few side-effects. With higher inhaled doses side-effects may increase, but simultaneous use of nonsteroidal agents (such as cromolyn or nedocromil) can lessen the side-effects. "Fear of side-effects should not deter asthmatics from using this medication," stresses one specialist. *"Unstable or severe asthma is far more dangerous."*

Bronchodilators remain an integral part of asthma management, but they are now used on an "as needed" basis to ease immediate breathing problems. Bronchodilators swiftly widen narrowed airways and ease labored breathing, but they do nothing to reduce the lung inflammation, which leaves the person open to fresh attacks. "Bronchodilators shouldn't be needed more than about twice daily," notes one specialist, "and they're best reserved for blunting flare-ups, not for regular use." If you are using bronchodilating drugs more than twice (or a maximum of four times) a day, you should seek further medical advice.

New classes of drugs being explored include mediator

blockers (for instance, leukotriene antagonists) to reduce bronchospasm; some of these are already on the market.

A Summary of the Main Anti-asthma Medications

Anti-inflammatory agents ("preventers")
- steroidal anti-inflammatories – e.g., budesonide (Pulmicort), fluticasone (Flovent), beclomethasone (Beclovent)
- nonsteroidal anti-inflammatories – e.g., cromolyn (Intal), nedocromil (Tilade)

Bronchodilators ("relievers")
- short-acting beta-2 agonists such as fenoterol, terbutaline, procaterol, salbutamol
- longer-acting beta-2 agonists such as salmeterol (in Canada), albuterol (in the U.S.)
- anticholinergic substances such as ipratropium
- xanthine (caffeine-like) compounds such as theophylline
- mediator blockers such as zafirlukast

Anti-inflammatory Agents
These medications reduce inflammation in the bronchial

Overuse of bronchodilators may lead to trouble

It's widely believed that bronchodilators are overused. Studies show that over-reliance on these drugs may in fact worsen asthma, because they open up the airways and allow in more irritating triggers. While the troubled breathing and shortness of breath may subside within minutes of taking a bronchodilator puff, the airway inflammation remains – leaving the risk of a severe attack. Indeed, bronchodilators may *mask* worsening lung inflammation, so that people are unaware of the seriousness of the problem – or deny it – and suddenly find themselves in a crisis situation, unable to breathe, and have to rush for emergency assistance. One New Zealand researcher linked increased asthma deaths among the Maoris to overuse of bronchodilators.

tissues and decrease mucus production, but can take time to work. Inhaled corticosteroids take some weeks to exert their anti-inflammatory effects, starting after 24 to 48 hours and usually peaking only after two to three weeks of use. Corticosteroids come as low- and high-concentration products, and as inhalers or tablets. Some physicians first prescribe non-steroidal forms, moving to steroidal anti-inflammatories for worsening or persistent cases. Very severe cases may require a short course of oral corticosteroids.

Steroidal anti-inflammatories

- *Inhaled corticosteroids* include beclomethasone (Beclovent), budesonide (Pulmicort) and fluticasone (Flovent). People may start out on 8 to 12 puffs a day to bring their asthma under control, and later taper to less – 2 to 4 puffs daily.

    Side-effects from inhaled corticosteroids are common but minor in adults on the usual doses, and may include *dysphonia* (voice hoarseness) and a mild fungal (yeast) mouth infection known as "thrush," or candidiasis – usually preventable by inhaling the drug before a meal, using a spacer device, or rinsing the mouth with water or gargling after inhaling the medication. Consult a physician about changing the dose if symptoms worsen or change.

- *Oral steroids* (such as prednisone) are required for severe asthma and emergency situations. People with severe asthma may need steroid tablets from time to time, often as a two-week course. Some asthmatics at risk of severe episodes keep tablets on hand at home in case of need – for instance, with a cough, cold, flu, sinusitis or bronchitis – and use them as well as the usual steroid puffer, stopping the tablets when the symptoms ease up. Steroid tablets are usually taken at breakfast-time to mimic the body's own natural rhythm of corticosteroid release. If you are on steroid tablets, inform any medical caregiver or dentist that you use them, and wear a medical-alert bracelet listing the condition you take them for.

Nonsteroidal anti-inflammatories

- *Cromolyn*, or *cromoglycate* (Intal), one of the safest anti-asthma drugs, comes as a metered-dose inhaler or in powder form, and is used as a preventive for regular control, rather than for quick breathing relief. It's especially useful in children with mild asthma (given from a nebulizer), and for exercise-related asthma (taken 10 to 20 minutes before starting a workout). But unfortunately it's not effective in all asthmatics.
- *Inhaled nedocromil* (Tilade), more powerful than cromolyn, is very effective in reducing an asthmatic cough, although not as effective as the new high-dose steroids. Again, it doesn't work in all asthmatics.
- *Oral ketotifen* (Zaditen) is a mild, "user-friendly" anti-inflammatory agent, often more helpful in children than in adults.

Bronchodilator "Quick-fix" Medications

Bronchodilators rapidly open up the airways by relaxing the smooth muscles encircling them, giving dramatic relief within minutes. Short-acting forms are used as needed, mainly as "rescue" medications to ease breathing discomfort, and are taken alongside regular anti-inflammatories. Long-acting forms are used for more severe asthma and may be advised for some asthmatics as "add-on" drugs, to be taken regularly as well as anti-inflammatories.

Beta-2 agonists (also called beta-2 adrenergics)

- *Short-acting inhaled beta-2 agonists* such as terbutaline

(Bricanyl), salbutamol (Ventolin) and procaterol (Pro-Air) relieve breathing within minutes of being inhaled. Beta-2 agonists are best used only as needed to ease breathing, not on a routine basis. It's wise to keep tabs on the number of bronchodilator puffs used daily to tell how well the asthma is doing. If beta-agonist puffs are needed more than usual – usually two to four times a day – the asthma is getting out of control, and it's time to seek further medical advice.

- *Long-acting beta-2 agonists* include salmeterol (Serevent). These have bronchodilating effects that last up to 12 hours, and may be helpful as "add-on" drugs, used as well as anti-inflammatories, for hard-to-control cases, especially if there's nighttime discomfort. Careful instruction is needed on their use, as well as close monitoring. They should not be used as substitutes for fast-acting forms, as they take a while to work, though they then give longer relief. They are not indicated for unstable asthma.

  Side-effects include tremors and rapid or irregular pulse. If the side-effects are annoying, consult your physician or an asthma clinic.

  Owing to emerging concerns that regular use (or high doses) of beta-2 agonists can worsen asthma or increase the risk of heart-rhythm problems, these drugs should only be used *when and as needed*, not regularly. Consult a physician about their correct use, especially if you need puffs more than two or three times a day.

Anticholinergic bronchodilators
- *Ipratropium bromide and oxytropium* are inhaled drugs that work on different (cholinergic) receptors than beta-2 agonists, and act more slowly. They are often combined with a beta-2 agonist to enhance airway dilation. For

example, ipratropium (Atrovent) may be given together with Ventolin to ease breathing. Side-effects are rare but may include mouth dryness and vision blurring.

Xanthine compounds
- *Theophylline and aminophylline bronchodilators* (e.g., Uniphyl, Theolair, Theo-Dur), taken as pills or syrups, are second-line airway dilators, now used less often. Theophylline can interact with some other drugs and various illnesses, so that its effects are distorted – for instance, viral infections, heart and liver diseases, and antibiotics and ulcer medications (e.g., cimetidine) may increase theophylline levels in the blood. Smoking, phenobarbital, phenytoin and high-protein diets decrease blood theophylline levels. These interactions, as well as side-effects such as nausea, diarrhea, headache, insomnia and tremors, are a frequent problem and theophylline use must be carefully monitored.

Mediator blockers
Since mediator chemicals cause many of the inflammatory changes in asthma, mediator antagonists are being developed, and one, zafirlukast (Accolate), taken as tablets, is already on the market in the U.S. and will soon be available in Canada. Its efficacy remains to be proven, and interactions with other drugs may prove troublesome.

The Hardware of Asthma Drugs
The best way to deliver asthma drugs is by inhalation through the mouth; this puts the drugs directly into the lungs, achieving an effect similar to that of oral medications at far lower doses, with fewer side-effects. There is now a wide range of inhalers to choose from, including metered-dose inhalers (MDIs); these may be pressurized with gas (pMDIs), or dry powder systems. There

Asthma Medications

Generic name	Some brand names	Action
Inhaled corticosteroids: "preventive" medications		
Beclomethasone	Beclodisk†, Becloforte (high dose), Beclovent, Vanceril	anti-inflammatory – reduces bronchial (lung) inflammation, decreases mucus; peak effects after 1–2 weeks; dampens underlying cause of asthma
Budesonide	Pulmicort, Rhinocort (in nose)	strong anti-inflammatory – same as above
Flunisolide	Aero-Bid, Bronalide	same as above
Fluticasone	Flonase (in nose), Flovent (in mouth)	anti-inflammatory – reduces lung inflammation; very effective; few side-effects
Triamcinolone	Azmacort, Kenacort*, Kenalog	reduces bronchial (lung) inflammation, decreases mucus; peak effects after 24–48 hours or more
Oral steroid tablets		
Dexamethasone	Decadron	anti-inflammatory; reduces airway inflammation
Methylprednisolone	Medrol	strong anti-inflammatory and powerful dampener of bronchial inflammation; decreases underlying cause of asthma; peak effect in 24–48 hours; side-effects of oral steroids may include face puffiness and weight gain, bone loss (with long-term use)
Prednisolone	Delta-Cortef, Pediapred, Prelone*	same as above
Prednisone	Deltasone, Meticorten*	same as above
Nonsteroidal anti-inflammatories		
Cromolyn (also called cromoglycate)	Intal, Nalcrom	mast-cell stabilizer and anti-inflammatory; tablets or nebulizer/ spray/powder; reduces inflammatory effect of mediators released by mast cells
Ketotifen	Zaditen (liquid or tablets)	antihistamine and mild anti-inflammatory; more useful for children than for adults
Nedocromil	Tilade	anti-inflammatory; blocks release of inflammation-causing mediators

*Available in U.S. only
†Available in Canada only

Asthma Medications (continued)

Generic name	Some brand names	Action
Bronchodilators (beta-2 agonists): "quick relief" medications		
Albuterol (in U.S.), salbutamol (in Canada)	Proventil*, Ventodisk†, Ventolin	fast-acting bronchodilator; use "as needed" for acute symptoms to relieve breathing problems; widens airways briefly; short-acting
Bitolterol	Tornalate	same as above
Fenoterol	Berotec	widens airways, relieves bronchospasm briefly (fast-acting)
Metaproterenol (in U.S.), orciprenaline	Alupent, Metaprel*	short-acting bronchodilator
Pirbuterol	Maxair	same as above
Procaterol	Pro-Air†	short-acting relief
Terbutaline	Brethaire*, Bricanyl†	short-acting bronchodilator; good for children
Bronchodilators (beta-2 agonists): slow-acting medications		
Salmeterol	Serevent	prolonged action
Anti-cholinergic drugs (inhaled)		
Ipratropium	Atrovent	slow-acting bronchodilator; dilates airway, clears lung obstruction and mucus; good for infants and elderly
Oxitropium	Oxivent*	same as above
Xanthine compounds (tablets)		
Aminophylline	Phyllocontin, Somophyllin*	mild, short-acting bronchodilator; slow-release airway widener
Oxtriphylline	Apo-Oxtriphylline†, Choledyl	short-acting bronchodilator
Theophylline	Pulmophylline, Quibron-T, Theo-Dur, Theolair, Theophyl, Uniphyl	mild, long-acting bronchodilator – slow airway widener, but considerable side-effects at excess dose (e.g., stomach upsets, nausea, headache, nervousness, insomnia); interacts adversely with some other drugs
Mediator blockers		
Accolate	Zafirlukast (tablets)*	leukotriene antagonist – blocks mediator (leukotriene) effects in narrowing airway

*Available in U.S. only
†Available in Canada only

are various add-ons, such as spacers (aerosol-holding chambers) and nebulizers (which spray in wet droplets through a mask). Some inhalers are easier to use than others. For maximum effect, learn to use your chosen inhalers correctly, follow package instructions and remember that cold temperatures and humidity reduce their efficacy. (Keep the inhalers warm and dry!)

Pressurized Metered-Dose Inhaler

1. Remove cap.

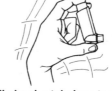

2. Shake the inhaler vigorously.

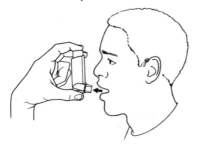

3. Hold the inhaler 1–2 inches (2–5 cm) from mouth (or put between lips), and breathe out normally (i.e., not a forced breath).

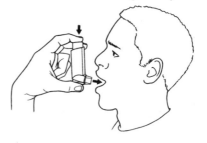

4. Tilt head back, breathe in deeply through mouth and push down on the metal inhaler top, releasing one puff of medication. Hold breath for 5–10 seconds, then breathe out.

Studies suggest that all too many asthmatics miss out on the maximum benefits of their medication because they don't use the inhalers correctly, or don't bother to try new types. (Ask your physician or a pharmacist for a lesson.)

The aim is to put as much of the drug as possible right into the lungs, leaving as little as possible in the mouth and throat. Many of the older devices leave almost 80 percent of the drug in the throat, and too little reaches the lungs. Some metered-dose inhalers are propelled by pressurized gases, and it's essential to coordinate the puff of medication with your breathing in. These inhalers also need time to recharge between puffs. Trial and error can show which inhaler works best for you. Many of the newer puffers with spacers require less meticulous timing. The addition of spacers (holding chambers) also improves drug delivery to the lungs.

Spacers (e.g., the Aerochamber) are a new development to ease drug delivery, avoiding the need to activate the inhaler and breathe in simultaneously. The inhaler is inserted into a

Aerochamber Inhaler (with Spacer)

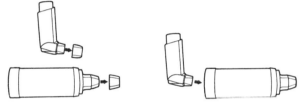

1. Remove cap from both inhaler and spacer.

2. Insert inhaler mouthpiece into spacer opening.

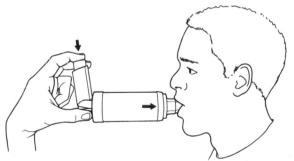

3. Shake well and breathe out; then put spacer mouthpiece into mouth and close lips around it.
4. Press down on metal canister of inhaler first, then breathe in through mouth deeply and slowly.

5. Hold breath as long as comfortably possible (about 10 seconds) while removing spacer.

tube-like device and the drug is released into the holding chamber; first you spray, then you inhale. Since breathing needn't be as carefully timed, people who have difficulty with standard pMDIs can use their drugs more effectively. Spacers added to pMDIs also help reduce side-effects such as sore throat, hoarse voice and yeast infections.

Dry powder inhalers are another advance. They use dry powder aerosols, and require just a small click to release the drug before you inhale it by suction. The powder inhalers are easy to use and to carry. The Rotahaler and Diskhaler deliver salbutamol – albuterol in the U.S. – (Ventolin) and beclomethasone (Beclovent); the Spinhaler is used for cromolyn (Intal), and the Turbuhaler delivers terbutaline (Bricanyl) and budesonide (Pulmicort). One disadvantage of powder puffers is that during a bad attack it can be hard to suck enough drug into

Turbuhaler (powder inhaler)

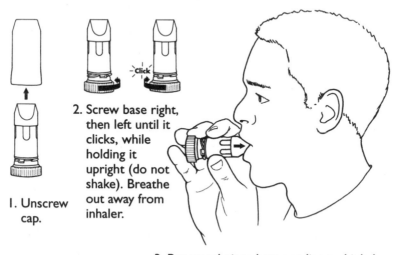

1. Unscrew cap.

2. Screw base right, then left until it clicks, while holding it upright (do not shake). Breathe out away from inhaler.

3. Put mouthpiece between lips and inhale deeply and forcefully through mouth. Remove puffer and hold breath for at least 5 seconds. Repeat as instructed. Clean mouthpiece 2 to 3 times a week as instructed.

Nebulizer

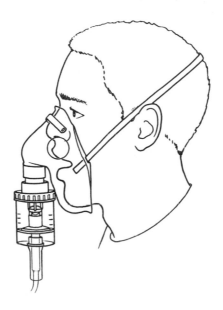

the lungs. Also, these inhalers do not reduce the throat irritation as much as spacers, since a fair amount of medication still ends up at the back of the throat and on the vocal cords.

Nebulizers use compressors, electrical or battery-powered delivery systems, to help deliver the drug. They produce a fine mist of droplets to be inhaled through a mask. They are useful for people unable to manipulate a metered-dose inhaler or spacer, such as young children and the elderly. They are also useful for severe attacks, but are bulky to carry and require a power source to activate them.

The right kind of drug delivery device depends on your personal preference and what you find easiest to use. Once you are used to a certain inhaler you may be reluctant to change, but consider trying some of the alternatives; it may well prove worthwhile.

Taking Control with an "Action Plan"

To gain optimal control over your asthma, work out an individual treatment plan, which includes an "action plan" for severe or worsening episodes, with your physician or other caregiver. You should be able to recognize worsening symptoms, and know what to do about them and when to get emergency aid. Therapy varies from one asthmatic to another, but the goal is to devise a treatment plan that lets you

- lead a normal life;
- have no (or minimal) wheezing, coughing and shortness of breath;
- avoid nighttime flare-ups, so you're not awakened by symptoms;
- exercise at will;
- require bronchodilators only occasionally;
- achieve good expired-air-flow rates and know when to step up treatment if flow rates fall;
- avoid severe episodes;
- recognize the early signs of a worsening attack, and deal with the problem, or get medical aid.

The first step in achieving control is to identify and try to avoid the triggers that set off your attacks. Some triggers can be modified; others must be accepted and lived with. Eliminating the source of the trouble can go a long way toward clearing up the symptoms. For example, smoking asthmatics should give up tobacco; those allergic to an animal may have to give away a pet. Those exceptionally sensitive to dust mites may be helped by creating as dustfree a living environment as possible.

Regardless of their best efforts to avoid triggers and create a non-asthmatic, allergen-free environment, many asthmatics require medication. Different doses and combinations of anti-inflammatories and bronchodilators are tried, often starting with anti-inflammatory treatment to reduce the need for bronchodilators.

Many specialists now believe that all asthmatics who experience daily symptoms should be treated with inhaled anti-inflammatories as well as bronchodilators. The latest treatment approach is based on the idea of asthma as a continuum, with drug therapy altered and tailored to match its changing severity. Severity is judged by the frequency and duration of symptoms, the extent of air-flow reduction and the amount of medication needed for control. In well-managed asthma, air-flow rates should remain near normal.

Signs of severe or badly controlled asthma

- nighttime symptoms
- a near-fatal episode, hospitalization or emergency-room visit for an attack
- decreasing morning air-flow (PEFR, or peak expiratory flow rate) measurements
- FEV (forced expired volume in one second) less than 60 percent of normal

Peak Flow Meter

1. Check that gauge is at zero.
2. Hold meter horizontally near mouth.
3. Take a deep breath.

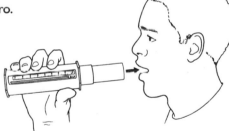

4. Seal lips around mouthpiece and breathe out as hard and fast as possible (a "fast blast" of exhaled air).
5. Read scale on gauge.
6. Reset and repeat twice.
7. Record best of 3 readings.

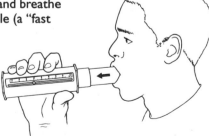

Note: Severe symptoms and greatly reduced air-flow rates call for an immediate burst of oral or intravenous steroids.

Measuring Air-Flow Rates Helps You Take Charge
Managing your asthma means watching for worsening symptoms, keeping tabs on changes in your lungs' air-flow rates and altering your medications accordingly. Airway blockage can build up and air flow can be diminished days before the worsening of the condition becomes noticeable in shortness of breath, more coughing or increased wheeziness. Therefore, if you can manage it, it's a good idea to keep tabs on your airways by using a peak flow meter.

A peak flow meter is a small, portable device to measure peak expiratory flow rates (PEFR) and determine how well air is being expelled from the lungs. It's easy to use and gives an objective assessment of lung blockage, independent of your actual symptoms – which may not yet portray the reality of a worsening situation – helping you know whether and when to increase your medication. If your airway blockage worsens, the measured flow rates will be below expected levels, even though you may not yet have noticeably worse symptoms. Detecting deteriorating lung function by this simple test can let you increase your medication when you need to, according to your action plan, maybe averting a severe attack.

To use the peak flow meter, check that the gauge is at zero. Hold the meter horizontally, take a deep breath, seal your lips over the mouthpiece and breathe out as fast as possible for one to two seconds. Read the gauge level, reset it and repeat the test twice. Record the best of the three readings on a chart.

Education Is As Vital As Asthma Drugs
Asthmatics often get into trouble because they lack knowledge about their disease, deny their need to take medications and fail to stick to their prescribed regimens. Many people with asthma

think their condition is "just an irritation" or can be treated with cough syrups, antibiotics and extra bronchodilator puffs. Studies show that teaching asthmatics to use their medications correctly, recognize danger signals and monitor their own air-flow rates can greatly improve their management of the condition.

"The chief strategy to reduce the toll of asthma," explains the head of one large asthma unit, "is education and more education – for patients, their families and sometimes also their primary-care providers." Surveys show that asthmatics who are conscientiously taught about their disease and the role and value of medications achieve far better control than those who get no guidance. "Bad outcomes could be prevented," notes one asthma expert, "if the symptoms were treated at once, and if people knew how to recognize the signals that herald severe asthma."

Exercise-induced Asthma

Exercise precipitates attacks in many asthmatics; indeed, some *only* wheeze following intense exercise such as jogging, jumping, skipping or playing hockey or football. Those predisposed to asthma usually find it harder to exercise in cold, dry air than in warm, damp conditions. Swimming rarely provokes attacks because the inhaled air is warm and humid. Most exercise-induced asthma comes on within a few minutes of starting the exercise, and it's usually short-lived, provided the person rests when short of breath.

Having asthma certainly doesn't mean that you should avoid activity. The more physically fit you are, the more efficiently your airway functions during exercise. Although there is no proof that any specific exercise improves or prevents asthma, regular activity to upgrade physical fitness is just as desirable for asthmatics as for other people.

A couple of puffs from a bronchodilating inhaler a half-hour before exercising can often prevent an attack. A recent study showed that inhaled cromolyn plus a beta-agonist bronchodilator is more effective in preventing exercise-related asthma than either drug alone. Many asthmatic athletes have relied on medication to permit them to participate in sport. But some anti-asthma stimulants are prohibited by sport doping laws, and a U.S. Olympic swimmer lost his medal in 1970 because he'd taken anti-asthma medication.

Asthma in Children

Asthma is the most common chronic childhood disease, affecting as many as 7 to 15 percent of children aged three to six. Many children continue to have episodes of varying severity up to their late teens. Children may have a first asthma attack at age three or four, but it can also start as early as six months, when it's often misdiagnosed as croup. While asthma in children resembles the adult form, it has some special features – particularly its similarity to "wheezy bronchitis," or recurrent chest infections, for which antibiotics may be prescribed; these do nothing for the asthma.

Persistent coughing is often the most common sign of childhood asthma, but it can be hard to distinguish the disease from recurrent colds. Telltale clues to asthma are unusually frequent colds followed by a cough that drags on for weeks, coughing that awakens the child at night, coughing a lot in daytime, several bouts of wheezing a year, noticeably labored breathing, coughing and wheezing after exercise and perhaps accompanying eczema. The condition has been defined by one expert as "three or more episodes of wheezing and shortness of breath – unless other causes are found." A child prone to frequent chest colds, a dry cough (especially one that worsens in the early dawn hours) and periodic breathing difficulties may well have asthma, and should be checked. Tests can often determine whether there are identifiable allergic triggers that might be eliminated or avoided.

Childhood asthma tends to be mild, with sporadic wheezing and/or cough, and can often be well controlled by no more than twice-daily bronchodilator puffs. Additional treatment is needed for children who wheeze with exercise, or on exposure to cold, dust mites, animals or other triggers. About 20 percent of asthmatic children have moderate disease, with episodes every four to six weeks. They may be started on nonsteroidal puffers – perhaps inhaled cromolyn or nedocromil – or on ketotifen (Zaditen) tablets or syrup.

If this doesn't keep symptoms down after a few weeks (longer in very young children), an inhaled corticosteroid may be suggested. The 5 percent or so of asthmatic children who have a severe problem, with breathing trouble on most days that's serious enough to interfere with school and sleep, need regularly inhaled corticosteroids plus bronchodilators for "breakthrough" wheezing. There are some concerns about steroids stunting children's growth, but newer inhaled agents are less likely to do so because the usual doses (50 micrograms per puff, no more than eight puffs a day) are only minimally absorbed into the bloodstream. Children on high doses should be monitored by a physician.

Good control allows young asthmatics to attend school and enjoy the usual childhood activities. However, treating asthma in young children can be hit and miss because of the difficulty of diagnosing the disease and administering medications, especially to infants. A spacer device or an Aerochamber with a mask may be the best way to give medication.

However, misconceptions about asthma being a "psychological condition," and fears or parental guilt about the condition, can hamper good management. Children themselves are often ashamed at having to use a puffer or take medicines in front of classmates. Tact and understanding are essential. The best advice is to try to treat the child as normally as possible, encouraging participation in all usual activities while carefully monitoring the condition. Charting breathing changes can be helpful, and keeping inhalers near obvious everyday items (such as a toothbrush holder) can help ensure that medications are taken regularly and not forgotten. Counseling asthmatic children and their caregivers can help youngsters not to feel undermined, stigmatized or handicapped by their breathing problems. Teachers and school staff can help by encouraging the children to participate as fully as possible, and by not calling them lazy or unmotivated if they have to restrict their sports activities. Using an inhaler before exercising may help.

Asthmatic teenagers are notoriously tough to manage because of their tendency to deny the existence of any problem, and their feelings of immunity and invulnerability, combined with their sense of insecurity and perhaps depression – which need to be recognized, understood and faced. Because they're apt to deny or ignore breathing problems and get into severe asthma attacks, adolescents are at particular risk. The persistent but erroneous belief that children outgrow asthma may lead to further neglect in recognizing and treating adolescent asthma. Children do *not* usually outgrow asthma, although they may come to have milder or minimal symptoms. Specialized counselors and "hot lines" open to adolescents can be helpful. For more on coping with asthmatic children, see Chapter Eight.

Coping with Nighttime Asthma

When asthma worsens, attacks also tend to increase at night

There's no magic climate

Asthma is as common in warm, dry climates as in wet, cold ones, so moving won't necessarily help. There's no way to predict whether your symptoms will be relieved except by spending a trial period in your proposed new residence. If allergens play a significant role, moving to a zone free of the relevant irritant – perhaps at higher altitudes – may minimize your symptoms. On the other hand, new environmental sensitivities may emerge!

("nocturnal asthma"), especially in the predawn hours ("morning dipping"). Like everyone else, asthmatics have a circadian (daily) rhythm in their breathing, and even normal airways tend to be narrowest between four and five a.m. – when body temperature and certain hormone levels are at their lowest. Being awakened by asthmatic discomfort two or more nights in a row is a warning sign to increase your medication, possibly to start on a long-acting bronchodilator as part of your personal action plan.

The Baffling Rise in Asthma Severity and Deaths

Yesterday's generation considered asthma a relatively mild disorder, and paid little attention to its potential severity. This attitude is becoming obsolete as more people develop asthma in their teen and adult years. Not only are more young people being diagnosed with asthma, but complacency about its "harmless" nature has been shattered by a steep rise in hospital admissions, emergency-room visits and deaths, especially during the 1970s.

The incidence of asthma has risen steadily since the early 1970s, and deaths have almost doubled in the past 14 years in many industrialized countries, although they are now leveling off in many places, including Canada and the U.S. For every asthma death there are hundreds of cases needlessly out of control, requiring better therapy. These figures don't mean that asthma is a common cause of death, even for asthmatics; but because asthma deaths are almost always preventable, the figures are far too high. While deaths from asthma remain rare, those who die have often had prior warning of their problems – previous life-threatening episodes, recent hospitalization for a severe attack, poorly controlled symptoms or having to go on oral steroids.

Exactly why more people are dying of asthma, not only in North America but also in Britain, New Zealand and other countries, remains a mystery. However, some reasons have been proposed for the upturn. One is that the condition is being more accurately and more frequently diagnosed, and is showing up more often as a cause of death on death certificates. Urban air pollution is another suspected reason – the increasing levels of ozone, sulfur dioxide, free radicals and other pollutants. But arguing against this theory is the fact that New Zealand – which has less polluted air – has more asthma deaths per capita than many more industrialized nations.

Other suggested reasons are diets rich in animal fats (a very speculative theory), and the increase in allergies and modern sealed buildings with carpets and soft furnishings, which expose people to high levels of indoor pollutants and airborne allergens. Allergens are key suspects, chief among them being molds, dust mites, cockroach antigens and animal dander. The finger is pointed at dust mites in particular because the introduction of mite-infested Western blankets into New Guinea led to an increase in asthma. So perhaps – for asthma as for allergies – the answer is to dust-proof the house and banish pets.

Another key reason thought to contribute to the rise in asthma deaths is the fact that people don't receive enough treatment, or the right treatment, in time – through their failure to follow the prescribed therapy, overreliance on airway-widening drugs and under-use of preventive anti-inflammatory medication, and the failure of physicians to recognize and treat the disease early and appropriately. Ironically, the availability of bronchodilating drugs may have magnified the danger, because these drugs widen the airways and give the asthmatic the sense that all is well even in the face of relentlessly progressing lung blockage.

Studies on deaths from worsening asthma show that patient and doctor alike underestimated the progress and severity of the attack, and failed to start aggressive treatment in time. Surveys in Britain, the U.S., New Zealand and elsewhere show that many people who died of asthma were given too little medication (e.g., corticosteroids), had received inadequate lung monitoring (which is simple to do, even at home) and were not followed up medically after severe episodes. Quite often, asthmatics wait for hours after using large amounts of their usual quick-relief bronchodilator before they seek medical aid, hoping that what works for a mild attack will ease a severe one. They may reach the emergency room too late, or even die en route to hospital.

Another suspected reason for the increase in asthma deaths is the fact that some asthmatics leave hospital too soon after medical treatment, without receiving proper medicines and instructions. Relapses or repeat attacks often occur shortly after a severe attack that wasn't adequately treated, especially in cases where the person should perhaps have been admitted to hospital but left before the asthma was fully stabilized. One British expert lists the "two absolute requirements for treating emergency asthma as measuring the extent of air-flow diminution, to check the extent of lung blockage, and immediate use of high-dose corticosteroids."

Recent North American guidelines for the emergency management of asthma also stress the value of measuring airflow rates, because while the observed symptoms – the amount of wheezing and shortness of breath – are an excellent indicator in some cases, they may not portray the full severity of an attack. *But the seriousness of symptoms should never be underplayed.*

"In emergency units we see two main kinds of severe asthma," explains one Canadian specialist in emergency medicine. "One is a rare, very severe, unexpected attack that can be fatal within hours – from hypoxia [oxygen lack] and cardiac arrest. The other, more typical case is someone with little understanding of the disease who allows a steadily worsening condition to grumble on for days, just taking more bronchodilator puffs, so the asthma goes downhill and the person ends up in emergency. Most of these cases recover well with correct treatment."

Hospital stays range from a couple of hours to several days, and treatment may include high doses of airway dilators given through a mask, careful air-flow monitoring, supplemental oxygen and corticosteroids – given by injection, through a mask or orally. Severe cases that respond poorly to emergency treatment may be admitted to hospital for a few days to stabilize the condition, to be sure the person isn't discharged too soon.

After a severe attack, people are often sent home with a course of corticosteroid tablets. "Any asthmatic sick enough to need emergency-department treatment," states one chief of a large emergency unit, "needs a short course of oral steroids." Education about asthma, and the prescription of oral steroids, can help prevent relapses.

Warning Signals of a Possible Emergency
While only a small proportion of asthmatics are at risk of life-threatening attacks, it's essential to know and heed the warning signals. Although some severe attacks strike "out of the blue," there are usually hints of impending danger – perhaps a previous acute attack, a need for hospital treatment that was taken too lightly, or too little instruction and follow-up.

Risk factors for a potentially severe asthma attack
- more than two previous emergency-room visits for asthma attacks
- having been admitted to hospital for a severe attack
- asthma requiring oral steroids
- recent withdrawal of oral steroids

Seek medical aid at once if you
- have symptoms not relieved by your usual medication
- need bronchodilators more than six times every 24 hours
- can't carry on your usual daytime activities
- notice deteriorating air-flow readings
- awaken from or are kept awake by asthmatic symptoms for several consecutive nights
- can't say a complete sentence without gasping for air

Risk factors that may precipitate a serious attack include respiratory infections, allergies, unrecognized deterioration in lung function, recent emergency-room treatment with short-lived improvement, noncompliance with prescribed therapy and misjudgment by both the physician and the patient of an attack's severity.

Never Deny the Problem or Delay Getting Help

People who delay seeking specialized help often do so because of unwarranted complacency (an assumption that the problem will go away), denial of their disease or reliance on people who can't recognize the dangers or provide life-saving assistance. Studies of children who died of asthma showed that denial and depression were common traits. *All asthmatics*, even those conscientiously following recommended treatment, should seek medical aid, call their physician or go to a hospital emergency department if they have signs of worsening obstruction.

Living with Asthma

While there is still no cure for asthma, it can be managed in a way that allows most people to lead a normal life. As one Toronto respirologist succinctly puts it, "Although the cause of asthma remains unknown, we can identify its triggers; although its mechanism isn't fully understood, we can measure its effect; and although there's no cure, it can be controlled." On a cautionary note, he adds that even people with mild or well-managed asthma must not be caught unawares by a severe attack. And when your condition is bad, he says, "don't get too despondent – it will get better and come under control, given proper treatment." Every asthmatic and his or her caregivers should learn about the disease, understand its possible severity and develop a treatment and action plan together with a knowledgeable, trusted healthcare provider.

Researchers are looking into the possible genetic underpinnings of this disease, with a view to prevention. Meanwhile, to help reduce acute attacks and control this very common disease, here are some principles we can follow to minimize the damage done by the disease.

- Thoroughly educate all asthmatics, and their families and caregivers, about the disease and its management, and make sure they get competent medical advice.
- Recognize that asthma differs from one person to another. Don't assume that what works for one person will necessarily suit others.
- Help asthmatics develop personal treatment and action plans in partnership with their physicians, and follow them.
- Promote the use of inhaled corticosteroids or other anti-inflammatories on a regular basis, especially if beta-2 agonist bronchodilators are often needed.
- Discourage the indiscriminate use of multiple drugs.
- Understand and promote the use of home peak flow meters to monitor changes in airways.
- Encourage asthmatics to improve the quality of their environment and lifestyle – for example, by reducing dust levels and avoiding tobacco smoke.
- Seek early medical assistance if it's needed – do not delay.
- Join, and promote the formation of, asthma support groups.

While all asthmatics have their ups and downs, most can obtain enough control to lead a normal life, given the advice of a competent caregiver who understands the disease. Do your best to find out as much as possible about the problem from the many organizations now available to offer help. (See the resource list at the end of the book.)

TEN

Food Allergies

Т**he subject of food allergy swirls with myths and mis-conceptions, and exaggerated views about the numbers of people affected. Although almost every food additive, coloring and other ingredient has been accused of causing "allergic" symptoms, food allergies are less commonplace than popularly imagined. Of the many adverse reactions to food first attributed to allergies, less than one-third turn out to be true allergic responses.

"Most of the adverse reactions to foods that bring people to doctors' offices," remarks one allergist, "are not allergies at all, but something else." Although accurate figures are hard to get, in North America about 3 percent of children (up to 8 percent in the first year of life) and roughly 1 percent of adults have a food allergy. Infants are more prone to food allergies because their immature immune systems react more strongly to "foreign" food proteins. (For more about children and food allergies, see Chapter Eight.) Some people die each year from allergic reactions to food, and many of the fatalities occur in people who also have other allergies, particularly asthma.

Distinguishing Allergy from Intolerance

Many people don't know how to distinguish between an allergic reaction and a food intolerance (such as lactose intolerance) or toxicity (such as food poisoning). While the symptoms of intolerance or toxicity may resemble those of an allergy, the causes, mechanism and treatment are very different.

Unlike food allergies, which can occur in minutes or seconds in response to a certain ingredient, an intolerance reaction usually involves larger amounts of food and takes longer (often hours) to appear. A person who develops a headache, gets irritable or feels edgy after consuming a particular food does not usually have an allergy. Someone who develops migraine after eating over-ripe cheese may be reacting to the tyramine in it; red wine also contains tyramine. This substance dilates blood vessels and may produce a headache, but that's not an allergic reaction. Chocolate, pineapple and citrus fruits – often accused of causing allergic reactions – rarely do. The phenylethylamine in chocolate may make people edgy and restless; strawberries and tomatoes are rich in histamine, and eating a large amount at once may cause some histamine-induced symptoms; but these are not true allergic reactions. Bacteria in undercooked beef may cause "hamburger disease," with vomiting, diarrhea and fever, but that's also not an allergic disorder.

Although there are some similarities – both allergies and food poisoning may cause stomach upsets and diarrhea – a true food allergy is a distinct and observable immune-system response to a specific food allergen (protein). Most food allergies involve the production of IgE antibodies and the release of mediators (such as histamine) from mast cells and basophils, and appear within 15 minutes at most; a few are delayed forms, involving a different immune mechanism, that surface 12 to 48 hours after the allergen is consumed.

It's surprising how many people are eager to blame what

ails them on what they eat, and especially on a food allergy, without any scientific backup. Although up to 40 percent of people *think* they are allergic to some food, only 3 percent suffer true immunological food reactions. Many people who are convinced that a certain ingredient makes them ill fail to react to it when skin-tested by allergists, or challenged with the suspected item hidden in the diet. For example, one woman claimed her headaches came from a sugar allergy, but when given a "challenge test" – fed sugar in an unidentifiable form – she failed to develop a headache. In another case, a woman convinced she was allergic to shrimps failed to show allergy symptoms when properly tested. If recognizable allergy symptoms cannot be reproduced by food-allergy testing, they stem from causes other than allergies.

A recent British study reported that one in five randomly selected households had members claiming to have a food allergy. The reported symptoms ranged from eczema, headaches and nasal problems to irritability, mood swings and hallucinations. Researchers investigating the validity of these claims found that only a tiny fraction of cases (less than 2 percent) were really allergies. The rest arose from a variety of non-allergic problems – food intolerances, aversions, gastronomic dislikes, metabolic deficiencies (such as lactose intolerance or phenylketonuria), diseases (such as cystic fibrosis), toxins, bacterial infections, eating disorders such as bulimia (deliberately throwing up to stay slim) and psychiatric problems (such as panic attacks).

A 1990 Toronto study illustrates some of the non-food-triggered symptoms commonly ascribed to foods. The researchers compared two groups of adult allergy patients, all of whom believed their symptoms were food-related. The people who complained of elaborate subjective symptoms such as memory loss, inability to concentrate, itchy earlobes, "pins and needles," sluggishness and sleep problems were not found to have food-triggered symptoms. Those with a *true* food allergy reacted to a food-challenge test with typical allergy symptoms – clearly visible hives, vomiting, swollen lips, tongue and larynx, facial flushing and a drop in blood pressure.

A few food additives, preservatives and colorings can also cause allergic reactions. For example, sulfites and metabisulfites are used as preservatives and "sanitizers" in sausage meats, salad dressings, beer, wine, coolers, and canned, frozen and dehydrated goods, and are added to salads and dried fruit to prevent spoilage and preserve crispness and color. Sulfites can provoke both intolerance and allergic responses, and people affected by them should seek the guidance of a licensed allergist – especially asthma sufferers, who are at particular risk of sulfite sensitivity. Despite restrictions introduced by the Food and Drug Administration in the 1980s, controlling their use in the U.S. on raw fruit, vegetables and fresh salads, the continued use of sulfites as food preservatives and anti-browning agents has come under increasing attack. In Canada, use of sulfites (including bisulfites and metabisulfites) is restricted but not banned. These additives may be found in such items as sliced fruit or vegetables, vinegar, jams, jellies and marmalade, pickles and relishes. Labels usually state amounts over 10ppm (parts per million) but some items are exempt from the labeling laws.

Complaints Widely Attributed to Foods, without Scientific Backup

- *mood changes* – anxiety, depression, weepiness, sadness
- *behavior or neurological problems* – hyperactivity, aggression, violence, criminality, bedwetting, temper tantrums; deep-rooted problems with many causes, requiring psychotherapy

- *vague malaise* – such as irritability, fatigue, an inability to concentrate. One man complained that fish made his skin "slimy and slithery" (a non-food problem that may indicate an underlying psychological disturbance)
- *colic in infants* – fussiness, irritability, intestinal pain, incessant crying – often blamed on a milk allergy, but rarely a true IgE-antibody-mediated reaction
- *migraine headaches* – possibly linked to food allergies, but the evidence isn't conclusive. Some foods may aggravate migraine via non-allergic mechanisms

Some Causes of Non-allergic Food Reactions

- *lactose intolerance* – an inherited deficiency of the enzyme *lactase*, required to break down lactose (milk sugar), which causes bloating and gastric discomfort. Lactose intolerance is common in Asians, Africans and populations that do not traditionally drink cow's milk
- *phenylketonuria (PKU)* – lack of the enzyme needed to metabolize the amino acid phenylalanine (necessary for growth and development). Children with this condition must have diets free of phenylalanine, to avoid mental retardation
- *celiac disease* – a delayed hypersensitivity in those who lack the metabolic ability to handle gluten from cereals (such as oats, wheat, barley and rye). Symptoms include diarrhea, bloating and cramps
- *favism* – a reaction to broad (fava) beans in people lacking the enzyme glucose-6-phosphate dehydrogenase, leading to fever, headaches and anemia
- *natural food toxins* such as those in green potatoes, aflatoxins in mold-contaminated products (peanuts, for example), inedible wild mushrooms, or oxalates in the leaves of rhubarb, sorrel and beet

- *monosodium glutamate (MSG) aversion* – also called "Chinese restaurant syndrome" – an intolerance of the MSG used as flavoring in some Chinese cooking and prepared foods. This leads to headaches, heart palpitations and numbness, and may exacerbate asthma
- *sulfite and metabisulfite intolerance* – adverse reactions (with a rash and/or wheezing), and occasionally severe asthma or anaphylaxis, as noted above
- *scromboid fish poisoning* – from spoiled fish containing a buildup of histamine
- *contaminated cheeses* (also with elevated histamine) – which can cause allergy-like "histamine poisoning"
- *sensitivity to natural pharmacological or druglike agents* in food. For example, caffeine in coffee, tea or colas can make some people jittery and anxious. Histamine in strawberries, blue cheese or eggplant can lead to headaches and flushing. Eaten in large amounts, the glycyrrhizic acid in licorice can raise blood pressure and enlarge the heart. Substances in certain spices (for example, nutmeg) can cause psychiatric symptoms
- *food poisoning* from improperly prepared or poorly stored food that becomes contaminated with bacteria. Examples include *salmonella* in eggs or *Campylobacter* in meat (such as hamburger), causing vomiting and diarrhea, usually several hours after the bacteria-laden food is eaten.

Food Allergies Are Immune-System Overreactions

A food allergy causes the body to produce excess IgE antibodies in response to harmless everyday foods. As with other allergies, the reaction does not usually occur on the first encounter with the food, but only after you have been sensitized to it, which can take several exposures. Once you are sensitized to a food, your immune system goes into action each time you eat that food. If you have an allergic reaction to a food you think you've never eaten before, it means you were *unknowingly* sensitized, possibly during infancy.

It's an enormous task for the immune system to keep tabs on harmful bacteria, viruses, parasites and other intruders and be ready to attack them instantly, meanwhile allowing through essential nutrients. Given that the average person ingests up to 100 tons (90,000 kilos) of food in a lifetime, it's surprising how few foods provoke the immune system into an allergic attack.

What happens is the same as with other type I allergies: IgE antibodies stimulate mast cells to release potent mediators such as histamine, which cause the allergic symptoms. The reaction can be incredibly swift and sometimes catastrophic – with red weals (hives) all over the body, tingling of the lips, swelling of the tongue and throat, a flushed face and troubled breathing, perhaps allergic shock and anaphylaxis. Immediate epinephrine injection is needed as an antidote.

Less often, a food provokes an allergy that is not type I; in that case the symptoms are usually less serious and tend to surface several hours later, or even a day or two after consumption of the allergy-provoking food, due to different immunological mechanisms.

Only a Few Foods Commonly Cause Allergies
A long list of foods – ranging from whitefish, cod and other fish, many crustaceans, nuts and buckwheat to sunflower seeds, kiwi fruit, mangoes, pinto beans, chestnuts and chamomile tea – are known to provoke allergic responses. Of food additives, only a few – such as sulfites and papain (a meat tenderizer) – have been linked to severe allergic reactions. However, while almost any food could cause an allergic reaction, only a handful commonly do so in North America, namely:

- eggs
- milk
- peanuts
- soy
- tree nuts
- fish
- shellfish
- wheat

Major food allergies vary from country to country, depending on the popularity of various foods. In Japan, children are often allergic to rice; in Scandinavia, where fish is common fare, fish allergies are frequent. Nobody quite knows why some foods are more allergy-provoking than others. In North America, the foods most notorious for causing severe anaphylactic reactions are peanuts (not true nuts but legumes), nuts (such as pecans, almonds, cashews), eggs and seafood – especially shellfish (such as crab, lobster, clams, oysters, crayfish, shrimp).

Oral Allergy Syndrome: Curious Cross-sensitivity

Oral allergy syndrome is a condition in which people allergic to one food or certain pollens "cross-react" to another plant or its fruit containing similar molecules. For example, if you have a pollen allergy you may cross-react when eating certain fruits and vegetables, developing an itchy mouth, nose and throat, swollen tongue and other symptoms. People allergic to ragweed pollen often get a tingly mouth on consuming cantaloupe or watermelon, or dandelions or chamomile tea (belonging to the same plant family). Those allergic to birch-tree pollen may react on eating several fruits (apples, cherries, peaches, plums, pears), and possibly also new potatoes and hazelnuts; and people allergic to mugwort pollen may itch on eating celery.

Although people with oral allergy syndrome usually suffer only mild symptoms, some develop severe reactions. Rarely, oral allergy syndrome results in anaphylactic shock. Some foods are less allergenic if processed or cooked. For example, people with birch-pollen allergy often react to fresh apples but not to applesauce, apple pie or apple juice. However, although fruits and vegetables with "heat-affected" allergens may be less allergenic if cooked or processed, other allergy provokers such as peanuts are not affected by cooking.

Besides cross-reactions between pollens and fruit, some people are cross-allergic to several biologically related foods. For instance, those allergic to one type of fish, shellfish or tree nut may develop similar symptoms if they eat other types of fish, shellfish or nuts. Someone allergic to cashews may also react to pecans, almonds, pistachios, walnuts and hazelnuts. One Baltimore allergist recommends that "once someone has had an anaphylactic reaction to a tree nut, extreme caution is advised in eating other nuts, unless challenge tests exclude cross-reactivity."

Similarly, people allergic to cod may develop symptoms on eating other fish – perhaps halibut, salmon, flounder and snapper. Swedish studies found that some children had multiple fish cross-reactivities while many did not. More studies on such cross-reactions are underway, to try to predict their likelihood, so that people don't need to shun a whole food class. It can be difficult, to say the least, for those allergic to a common food – say, milk or wheat – to shop, cook and ensure a healthy diet while avoiding such a commonplace ingredient. "Widespread dietary exclusions are rarely necessary," notes one U.S. allergist, "and every effort must be made to accurately diagnose a food allergy, in order to avoid overly constrained diets that could undermine health."

Recognizing a Food Allergy

Food allergy tends to be a systemic reaction involving the skin, gastrointestinal tract and respiratory system, but the symptoms vary according to the person and the provocative agent. The

Who is at risk of food allergy?

Reliable food-allergy statistics are few and far between. The best figures available are based on surveys done in the U.S. and Europe during the 1980s. In the U.S., severe or anaphylactic food reactions affect less than 1 percent of the adult population and deaths from food allergies are estimated at about 100 each year. However, more children – according to one U.S. study, as many as 8 percent of children under age three – may suffer from adverse reactions to foods, of which about 2 to 3 percent are allergic reactions. Studies done during the 1980s in the U.S., U.K. and Europe found 2 to 3 percent of infants allergic to cow's milk. Research suggests that there may be an inherited predisposition in some cases. Breastfeeding for as long as possible and delaying the introduction of solid foods in infancy may help to delay or mute childhood food allergies; see Chapter Eight.

first hint of an allergic food reaction – which often appears within minutes or seconds of eating the offending morsel – may include any of the symptoms listed below but is often a tingling, numbness or itching in the lips, tongue and mouth, followed by swelling of the throat and maybe nausea, cramps, projectile vomiting, wheezing and breathing problems.

Warning Signs of Food Allergy
- itching, tingling of tongue and lips
- upset stomach, nausea, vomiting (later, diarrhea)
- hives or rash anywhere on the body
- swelling of throat, larynx and tongue
- flushing
- wheezing, difficulty breathing
- sudden drop in blood pressure (weakness), shock
- sense of doom
- unconsciousness

Food Allergies and Anaphylaxis
Food-induced anaphylaxis is occasionally fatal, most often in

people who have already experienced a severe episode. In one study, the foods most often incriminated were peanuts, tree nuts, shellfish and fish. Another study, in 1992, looked at six fatal and seven near-fatal episodes among children and teens who unknowingly ate foods to which they were allergic – eggs, milk, peanuts and nuts. One of the children was rushed to hospital but discharged too soon, only to suffer a fatal "late-phase" attack some hours after. Although all the victims had suffered previous anaphylactic episodes, none was carrying an epinephrine self-injector. The fatalities occurred in public places far from medical aid and resuscitation equipment. Several of those who died had other underlying allergy-linked disorders, such as asthma.

Studies show that fatal and near-fatal anaphylactic attacks often happen away from home, when people eat something without realizing that it contains the allergen. The deaths are often linked to a denial of, or failure to recognize, the severity of the attack; not treating it promptly; or misguided reliance on antihistamines to relieve it. Experts stress that diligent avoidance of allergens, greater recognition of the risk and carrying an epinephrine self-injector kit are the best protection.

"To reduce the risk," says one expert in emergency medicine, "people who suffer an anaphylactic food attack must be kept under hospital surveillance for long enough after being revived with epinephrine. They should be observed for up to 12 hours after a severe attack, as symptoms can resurface in a second-wave reaction, possibly worse than the first." Corticosteroids may be given to offset a late-phase reaction. Before being discharged, they need to be informed of the severity of their condition, and advised to obtain nutritional advice and follow-up evaluation by an allergist. They should also be pre-scribed a self-injector kit.

Few people have multiple food allergies

The majority of food-allergic people react to only a few foods. However, people often think they are allergic to many foods and restrict their diet, needlessly curtailing the variety and pleasure of eating and perhaps also jeopardizing their health. For example, Mary, a 30-year-old, thought her diet was making her depressed, irritable and tired. Convinced that she was allergic to chocolate, sugar, most fruits, alcohol, lamb, fish, beef and dairy products, she avoided these items, rendering her diet unpalatable and boring. She had trouble eating in restaurants and her friends didn't invite her to dinner because she was so difficult to cook for. Mary was an extreme case, but many people believe that a wide variety of foods make them ill or undermine their health. Double-blind challenge tests show that individuals are rarely allergic to more than one type of food. The exceptions – those who have multiple food sensitivities – need expert dietary advice so that they eat properly and don't compromise their nutritional health.

Food-dependent, Exercise-induced Allergies

As noted earlier, vigorous exercise following a meal or after eating a specific food occasionally precipitates allergic symptoms – sometimes severe ones, even including anaphylaxis – hence the scientific term "food-dependent, exercise-induced anaphylaxis." This curious allergy was first linked to the ingestion of certain foods among athletes in 1974, and is now on the rise – perhaps because of increasing interest in jogging, aerobics and other fitness activities.

Exercising without eating beforehand does not cause allergic symptoms in these cases. The reaction only comes on if people exercise vigorously within 5 to 24 hours of eating, or of consuming a specific food – notably shellfish, fruit or celery. It usually starts with large hives, skin tingling and itching, flushing all over the body, swelling and faintness, generally lasting two to four hours. In severe cases there is difficulty breathing, vascular (blood system) collapse and anaphylaxis. Experts speculate that the combination of food and vigorous exercise somehow increases the mast cells' release of allergic mediators.

In one case, an allergy-prone woman collapsed with widespread hives and labored breathing whenever she exercised after eating peaches. In another, a Boston businessman found his palms and soles became itchy, and he broke out in hives, felt faint and couldn't breathe, whenever he exercised within two hours of eating dinner – but he had no reaction if he ate dinner without doing his daily five-mile run afterwards, or if he ran without eating beforehand. In another instance, a young college athlete, who frequently ate shrimp with no aftermath, developed large welts and intense itching when he did his daily workout soon after eating shrimp. Half an hour into his exercise routine, his face and tongue swelled up; he could hardly breathe and he felt faint. Fortunately, a physician at the sports clinic revived him with an epinephrine shot. In this case, neither exercise alone nor just eating shrimp brought on the reaction – it was the shrimp–exercise combination that caused trouble.

Recent reports have also incriminated chicken and wheat in food-dependent, exercise-induced anaphylaxis. Obviously the solution is to avoid the combination of allergy-provoking foods and exercise. Should an attack occur, treatment is the same as for any other form of anaphylaxis – epinephrine injection. Exercising with an informed companion is a wise precaution.

Diagnosing Food Allergies

Diagnosis depends on a full medical history, the described symptoms – when, where and how fast they occurred, whether the food was raw or cooked, eaten at home or out, how much food was needed to bring on the reaction – and many other details. In some cases it's easy to identify a food allergy. If your tongue starts to tingle, and your lips swell and hives appear, within minutes of swallowing a mouthful of lobster, the answer is simple: you're allergic to lobster. But diagnosing a food allergy can be tricky. Physicians must rule out the possible non-allergic causes – such as metabolic diseases (e.g., phenylketonuria or lactose intolerance), food toxins, infections, gastrointestinal disorders (such as ulcers or gallstones), drugs and eating disorders.

Skin or challenge tests may be done to try to pinpoint the offending food allergen, in a clinic or doctor's office with full emergency backup, in case of a severe reaction.

Skin prick tests are used to identify or confirm an IgE-mediated allergy to a specific food. Properly done, they are reproducible and are an excellent way to *exclude* a food allergy. A negative prick test – with no redness or swelling where the food was applied – is 95 percent reliable. In other words, if no weal and flare develop in someone suspected of a shrimp allergy, there is a 95 percent chance that the person is not allergic to shrimp. Skin prick tests are less good at *confirming* a food allergy. A positive response indicates less than a 50 percent chance that someone's symptoms arise from a particular food. Sometimes allergists try using fresh food (apple, celery, shrimp) because extracts are so unreliable. Thus prick tests are evidence to be interpreted in the light of the whole picture and the person's medical history.

Intradermal (deeper) skin testing increases the risk of producing a serious systemic reaction and is even less accurate, so it's rarely done.

Elimination diets may be tried to determine whether a food is producing allergic symptoms; prime suspects are totally eliminated from the diet for a few days and then added back one by one. If symptoms persist in the interim, these particular items cannot be blamed for the allergy. If the symptoms disappear and return when a certain food is added back, it means the food is likely creating the symptoms. This test is usually only used for non-life-threatening symptoms (such as hives). Elimination diets aren't considered reliable, and are not suitable for more than a week or two in children because of the risk of nutritional deficiency.

The RAST blood test, measuring food-specific IgE levels in the blood, is less sensitive but may be done when skin tests cannot be used or give dubious results. It proves that someone is sensitized to a certain food and has the IgE antibodies, but not that the food is sure to trigger symptoms, or what their severity would be.

Double-blind food challenge tests are the "gold standard" for confirming a food allergy, but must be done in a clinic or hospital setting in case of a severe response. Obviously, if someone breaks out in hives, has a swollen tongue or can't breathe each time a certain food is eaten, there's no need for challenge tests. But if the symptoms are vague and the offending food is unknown, or if skin prick tests give uncertain answers and there's doubt about what's causing the food allergy, a blind challenge may be tried; see Chapter Four. If the tests are all negative but symptoms persist, food is not likely to be the problem.

As an example of the unreliability of many allergy tests, take the case of an elderly man with an egg allergy who had a skin prick test with a number of foods, including eggs. His skin test was positive for eggs, as expected. However, it was also positive for milk. He was surprised because he had been drinking milk all his life without any problems. Nevertheless, the allergist urged him to give up milk. The man stopped drinking milk – a valuable source of calcium, protein and vitamins – impoverishing his already poor diet on the basis of a faulty skin-test result.

In contrast, consider three-year-old Nicky, from a highly

allergic family, who tested positive for peanuts in the skin-prick test although his parents were sure he had never eaten peanuts. The physician tentatively diagnosed Nicky as peanut-allergic, because he might have been sensitized to peanuts by some item such as a sauce or cookie containing peanuts or peanut products. The allergist recommended that Nicky avoid all peanut products for several years, at which time he could be retested. Better to be safe than sorry.

Managing Food Allergies

Since there is no cure or preventive treatment, avoidance is the only way to manage a food allergy – taking care not to eat or taste anything containing even traces of the offending ingredient. Despite the best of precautions, however, it's not always possible to completely shun the allergen. It may be present in some dish or prepared item. People allergic to common foods must be prepared for exposure to hidden allergens, and know what to do. Everyone known to have a severe food allergy should have on hand an epinephrine self-injector kit (see Chapter Five) for use at the first hint of breathing problems or other systemic symptoms. Denial of the severity of an attack, or failure to inject epinephrine in time, can have dire consequences. Although people with food allergies generally don't develop more severe reactions with each succeeding attack, this cannot be relied upon, and they must be prepared for worsening reactions.

Other life-saving measures given in hospital may include gastric lavage to clean out the stomach, oxygen, intravenous fluids to raise blood pressure, antihistamines, and corticosteroids to reduce the inflammation.

Desensitizing allergy injections have not been used for food allergies, although there are some very preliminary reports of the experimental use of "rush immunotherapy" to reduce the severity of peanut allergy. These studies have been inconclusive. Desensitizing allergy injections against food allergies are not currently recommended. More controlled studies are needed to show the efficacy and safety of such an approach.

Perpetual Need to Stand on Guard

Those with severe food allergies must be forever vigilant and on the lookout for allergens lurking in unexpected places. If you are allergic to some non-essential (although delicious) food such as lobster or oysters, having to avoid it may be annoying but it's not really burdensome. However, if you are allergic to a dietary staple such as wheat, milk or eggs, eliminating it from the diet needs careful planning.

Dietary counseling may help you ensure adequate nutrition, by suggesting good substitutes for nutrients you have to eliminate. Planning an allergen-free diet can be complicated, involving changes in cooking, shopping and meal preparation. Your allergist or family doctor can recommend a registered nutritionist able to give dietary advice.

Being Your Own Detective

Allergy-prone people must also become meticulous label readers and food watchers. Those at risk (or their caretakers) must learn to identify words used on food labels that indicate a "hidden ingredient" (see summary at end of chapter).

There are countless examples of the need to be on guard. When the lips of one egg-allergic man began to swell as he was drinking coffee in a café, he immediately questioned the server, and it turned out that the coffee had been passed through eggshells in the coffee percolator to keep it from tasting bitter. As another example, a Canadian resident allergic to milk developed a puzzling allergy to bread. On investigation, Health Canada discovered that milk had contaminated the bread at the manufacturing plant.

Never assume that a food or prepared dish is free of a dangerous allergen; always ask. Remember that an overzealous salesperson may give you the answer you seem to want; ask, "Is there shrimp in this?" rather than "There isn't any shrimp in this, is there?" Nor should a hostess think that a dinner guest sensitive to peanuts or eggs "just doesn't like them." The results could be tragic. Most people have heard stories about someone being rushed to hospital after eating an allergen that was not on the ingredient list, or that they were told was not included. Ingredient information is key to preventing adverse reactions, but accidents, although rare, have been known to happen. There can also be cross-contamination during food production, preparation or handling. Chocolate that drips off nut candies may be remelted and poured over non-nut candies; a few shrimp in a salad bar may become scattered in another ingredient.

Good news for Canadians with food allergies is that many restaurants will provide detailed ingredient information on menus. More than 1,800 restaurants, including nine national chains, are participating in the Allergy Aware Program, established by the Canadian Restaurant and Food Services Association. To date, no such program is reported across the U.S.

Never Forget Your Self-injector

Despite all precautions, people with food allergies may still unknowingly be exposed. Therefore, being prepared and knowing what to do are the best protection. The difference between a fatal and near-fatal allergy attack may depend on swift recognition of the emergency by an alert relative, friend or bystander, immediate injection of epinephrine and prompt summoning of medical aid. It's crucial not to wait until the person is obviously collapsing. Don't be lulled into a false sense of security because you've dealt with a severe reaction in the past. Remember the potentially fatal nature of anaphylaxis; never deny oncoming or early symptoms, but act *at once* and use the self-injector.

The EpiPen and Ana-Kit are available by prescription. It's also wise to wear a medical-alert bracelet or necklet naming your allergy. Even if symptoms abate swiftly after injection, proceed quickly (or have someone take you) to a hospital emergency department. Although your immediate symptoms may fade, late-phase symptoms can appear up to 12 hours later.

Oddly enough, many people at risk of anaphylaxis fail to carry the kit with them. In one tragic example, a woman allergic to eggs suffered three anaphylactic episodes during the four years she worked in a large office, each one requiring her boss to rush her to hospital. On the fourth attack she was alone in the office, and when her boss got back from his lunch he found her in a coma; by the time she reached hospital it was too late to save her.

The Peanut Problem

Peanut butter and other peanut products are being increasingly branded as "danger foods," because this allergy seems to be on the rise. Recent reports of severe peanut allergies (especially in children), even some deaths, have produced alarming headlines. But to put the "peanut panic" into perspective, having a peanut allergy does *not* mean danger around every corner, and an inevitably untimely death. What it does mean is that peanut-allergic people must manage their allergy safely, take care not to eat peanut-containing foods, keep tabs on what's consumed (especially away from home), carry an emergency kit and follow recommended guidelines.

"The key," comments one allergist, "is to respect, not fear, the peanut; know what it is and take proper precautions."

The peanut, *Arachis hypogaea*, is not a nut but a legume, related to beans, peas, soy and lentils. The plant is a bush with yellow flowers and a long stalk, and the pods holding the so-called nuts grow below ground. Cultivated since 2000 B.C., peanuts are favored for their amazing versatility: they can be eaten whole as snacks, crushed into paste, refined into oil and incorporated into countless foods. But peanut proteins can act as powerful allergens, even in tiny amounts, and emergency departments report that, of severe anaphylaxis cases coming into North American hospitals, one of the most common causes is peanut allergy.

However, not all peanut allergies are severe. Some cases are quite mild and just produce a face rash or a tingly tongue. "The problem is knowing whose peanut reaction will become more severe," notes one allergist. "At present, we have no way of predicting who's likely to have a severe, perhaps life-threatening episode the next time peanuts are eaten. So we have to treat all cases as potentially serious."

Many industrialized countries report a sharp rise in peanut reactions, with growing numbers of North American and European children testing allergic to this food, perhaps because they're exposed at ever younger ages to more and more peanut products. According to the American Peanut Council, U.S. peanut consumption averages 11 pounds (5 kilograms) per person per year, about half of it as peanut butter. First produced in the early 20th century as a cheap source of valuable protein, peanut butter is an increasingly popular childhood food. Almost 80 per cent of children have tasted it by their first birthday – before their immune systems are fully mature. In one study of 90 children, all had eaten a peanut-containing product before the age of two. Children may even be sensitized while breastfeeding, through traces of peanut in the mothers' breastmilk. Allergic sensitization may be increasing because of both the expanding diversity of peanut products and their consumption at younger ages.

In managing peanut allergy, *avoidance is the key* – not eating anything containing even traces of peanut – but it's also essential to carry an epinephrine self-injector in case of need, and to use it at the first hint of an attack. To protect children in allergy-prone families, parents are advised to withhold peanuts until the children are at least three years of age.

Peanut-allergic people must always be on guard for peanut traces. Peanuts are now used as ingredients in a vast array of cookies, pastries, candy, cakes, dips and sauces – especially in Thai, Vietnamese and African dishes – and even in Chinese eggrolls, where peanut butter may be used to seal the ends. Peanuts may be deflavored and reconstituted to mimic real nuts, such as almonds, walnuts or cashews. Peanut oil can be used in medications. Even a minute amount – a speck of peanut on the lips – can bring on a reaction. Eating food prepared with unwashed utensils or machines formerly used for peanuts is enough to trigger an attack. For example, a young girl recently had a near-fatal episode when she ate a chocolate ice-cream cone tainted with peanut from a previous scoop. Someone else died from eating peanut butter as a "secret ingredient" used to thicken a chili dish. Similarly, a young girl collapsed and died at a summer camp within minutes of eating a sandwich prepared with a knife bearing remnants of peanut butter.

Tips for Preventing and Managing Peanut Allergies

- *Do not feed infants born into allergy-prone families* peanuts or peanut butter until age three or later.
- *If breastfeeding an allergy-prone infant,* avoid eating

The push for peanut-safe classrooms

Many physicians are calling for "peanut-safe classrooms" in cases where an allergy-prone child is attending, as even scraps of peanut butter or peanut snacks can endanger a vulnerable child. "It cannot be stressed enough," notes one emergency physician, "that minute amounts of peanuts can be life-threatening. The number of anaphylactic episodes in schools is increasing, emphasizing the need for greater awareness."

Some schools have created "peanut-safe" classrooms, a few have forbidden peanut products anywhere on the premises and some experts have suggested a peanut ban in all daycare centers and kindergartens attended by peanut-sensitive children. However, the recommendation to ban or limit peanut products is controversial, as peanuts are good sources of cheap protein; also, forbidding children to eat peanut butter at school infringes on personal liberty and may be unduly restrictive. Critics also say that peanut bans may make children feel ostracized, or give them a false sense of security so that they're less vigilant. "Schools should be peanut-safe rather than peanut-free," suggests one allergist at Toronto's Sick Children's Hospital, "with certain classrooms excluding peanut products if necessary."

peanuts, to prevent sensitization through breastmilk.

- *Alert teachers, neighbors, school and daycare personnel* to the presence of a peanut-allergic child.
- *If there are known peanut-allergic children in the school,* try not to send peanuts, peanut butter or other peanut products to school, and consider peanut-safe classrooms.
- *Watch for hidden peanut,* especially hard to detect in items such as ice-cream, "veggie" burgers, cakes, gravy, cookies and Chinese, Thai, Vietnamese or African food.

Summing Up: Preventing and Controlling Food-allergic Reactions

- *Pay heed to early warning signs* (hives, nausea and vomiting) that may herald a food allergy.
- *Read food labels* with scrupulous care.

- *Read labels every time* you buy a product. (Ingredients may change.)
- *If you or a family member suspects a food allergy,* consult a physician or licensed allergist – don't try to treat yourself.
- *Get advice from a dietitian* to plan a nutritious diet that excludes allergenic foods.
- *Be wary when dining out.*
- *If you are asthmatic,* be extra careful; severe food reactions can precipitate a massive asthmatic attack.
- *Contact food companies* for ingredient information (the address or phone number is usually on the food label).
- *Wear a medical-alert bracelet* if you have a severe food allergy.
- *Carry a self-injector kit at all times,* if you are at risk of anaphylaxis; never leave home without it.
- *Breastfeed babies* for their first six months and withhold highly allergenic foods for their first two to three years.
- *Learn to decipher food labels.* By law, prepared foods should list ingredients, but the terminology can be tricky. Sometimes the presence of an ingredient is indicated by a related word:
    - for eggs look for "ovo-words" such as *ovomucin* and *ovalbumin*; also *globulin, albumin* and *lecithin*
    - for milk look for "lacto-words": *lactalbumin, lactoglobulin, lactose*; also *casein, whey, caseinate,* as well as cream, curds, butter, cheese
    - for peanuts watch for hydrolyzed vegetable protein, *NuNuts* (reconstituted nuts)
    - for wheat look for bran, flour, graham flour, farina, semolina, gluten, modified food starch
    - for soy look for miso, tamari, soya, vegetable protein, cereal, vegetable broth, vegetable gum, vegetable starch

- *Be cautious with unlabeled foods.* Many prepared foods are exempt from labeling requirements and need not list ingredients; for example, bakery products.
- *Know your ingredients.* Learn the dishes that are likely to contain the allergen in question; for example:
  - corn in tacos, tamales, tortillas, polenta, hominy grits
  - eggs in zabaglione, tiramisu, Caesar salad
  - milk in trifle, white sauce, custard
  - nuts in mincemeat, pesto, pâté, salad, marzipan
- *Watch for cross-contamination.* For example, a cook may butter bread with a knife previously used to chop eggs.
- *In a restaurant,* explain the problem and ask about the meal's ingredients.
- *Watch for cross-reactivity.* People allergic to certain items may also react to items of similar botanical classes, or with similar proteins; for example:
  - latex and certain foods, such as bananas, chestnuts, kiwi fruit and avocados
  - shrimp, crab, lobster and other crustaceans
  - tree pollens, especially birch pollen, and apples, cherries, celery; ragweed, and watermelon or cantaloupe; mugwort pollen, and celery
  - although peanuts and tree nuts were thought not to be involved in cross-reactions, recent studies show that some people with peanut allergy may also react to tree nuts (such as walnuts and pistachios)

  However, people allergic to eggs are not allergic to chicken; and people allergic to bee venom are not allergic to honey.
- *Speak up!* Be forthright, and inform friends, new partners and colleagues about your allergy. If you are asked out to dinner, explain – politely but frankly – what your allergy

is. On the other hand, if a guest advises you of an allergy, jot down the information in your address book for next time; your "good memory" will be appreciated!

ELEVEN

Insect Allergies

Most of us are all too familiar with the itchy red swelling or bumps caused by insect bites and stings. Scientists tell us that the average North American gets stung by an insect at least once every ten years, and bitten far more frequently. Many insects either bite or sting, but a few, such as some ants, are both biters and stingers. A local reaction at the sting or bite site is usual, and while it may itch, hurt and look ugly, it is usually gone in a day or two. Occasionally the discomfort lasts a couple of days, and the redness can linger for up to five days. Rubbing the site tends to worsen the swelling and can lead to a secondary infection.

Insect bites and stings sometimes produce very large, inflamed swellings, especially on the neck or face. But although localized insect reactions can be painful and look alarming, no special treatment other than ice packs is usually needed. If you have other symptoms, or if the inflammation worsens, contact your family physician. If the area develops an infection, antibiotics may be needed to clear it.

Some reactions to insect bites or stings are allergic in nature, and potentially far more serious. Allergic reactions to insect stings are caused by the venom injected into the skin through stingers; those from bites are a response to allergy-provoking substances (proteins) in insect saliva. If an insect sting or bite causes symptoms that extend beyond the local area to affect many parts of the body, it needs *immediate* medical attention. A systemic reaction may spread rapidly – within 10 minutes or so, but sometimes within seconds – through many body systems at once, leading to life-threatening allergic shock and anaphylaxis.

Allergic reactions to stings are usually more severe than those to bites. Experts estimate that for the North American population the risk of having a serious anaphylactic sting reaction is about 0.4 percent. In other words, almost one in 200 people is at risk of allergic shock from an insect sting. Stings in the neck and head region pose the greatest danger.

Once someone has had a severe, anaphylactic sting reaction there is a high likelihood of an equally bad, or worse, reaction to a further sting from the same type of insect. The shorter the time between the sting and the start of symptoms, the more severe the reaction is likely to be. But contrary to popular mythology, insect allergies do *not* necessarily worsen with each subsequent attack. Only about 5 to 10 percent of those who have a large local reaction go on to experience more severe, or even anaphylactic, reactions. Still, anyone with a history of severe insect allergy should wear a medical-alert tag, and ask an allergist about sensible precautions.

Stingers versus Biters

Fortunately, of the world's countless stinging insects, only a few commonly cause anaphylactic shock – in particular some of those in the order *Hymenoptera*, which includes the Apidae (honeybees, bumblebees and wasps) and Vespidae (yellow jackets, and yellow-faced, bald or white-faced hornets).

Some facts and statistics on insect attacks

- Every year about 50 North Americans die of allergies to insect stings.
- Insect stings most frequently causing anaphylaxis are those from yellow jackets, followed by bees, wasps and hornets.
- The enzymes (proteins) phospholipase and hyaluronidase are the main allergy-causing components in insect venom.
- The honeybee dies after it stings, but the wasp, hornet, yellow jacket and fire ant can sting repeatedly.
- Through "cross-reactivity," someone sensitized to yellow jackets may also be allergic to wasp and hornet stings.

Spiders too have been known to cause severe reactions. Harvester ants and fire ants – a recent wingless import into the U.S. – can deliver multiple, searing stings. But in North America, yellow jackets are most often responsible for severe insect reactions.

Biting insects such as fleas, mosquitoes, black flies, sand flies and ants tend to cause primarily local discomfort. However, insect bites (especially those of deerflies and horseflies) can occasionally trigger an anaphylactic reaction. Besides insect bites and stings, the feces of some insects (such as dust mites) and dried-up body parts of cockroaches, beetles, midges and some other insects can, when inhaled, cause allergic symptoms and exacerbate asthma in sensitive individuals; see Chapter Seven.

Who Is Most at Risk?

A serious, generalized allergic reaction to an insect attack sometimes occurs when someone thinks he or she has been stung for the first time, but in fact the person has almost certainly been sensitized (albeit unknowingly) by a previous exposure. A first episode is rarely fatal. In one study of 187 factory workers evaluated after insect bites and stings, 17 percent had large localized reactions, and 4 percent had significant generalized allergic reactions.

Most severe reactions and deaths from insect allergy occur in adult men. Adverse reactions are more common in boys than in girls, perhaps because boys tend to spend more time in outdoor activities. About 30 to 60 percent of adults who have suffered one serious insect reaction go on to have another. When they do occur, generalized allergic reactions usually begin within seconds to minutes of the insect sting, though occasionally they appear up to one hour afterwards.

"Since allergists cannot predict who is most at risk," notes one physician, "we recommend that everyone who has had a severe, generalized allergic insect reaction should always have on hand an emergency self-injector kit." Family members and friends should also know how to use the kit. If you know you're severely allergic to insects, try not to be alone outdoors so that others are around in case of need. Emergency kits should be replaced when they expire. (For more details about self-injector kits, see Chapter Three.)

Some people with severe sting allergies are candidates for venom immunotherapy, but they first need a thorough assessment by a competent allergy specialist.

Key Symptoms of Insect Allergy
In an already sensitized individual, the response to the insect

---

About insect stings

A stinging insect injects venom into its victim via a tiny, needle-like stinger on its posterior parts. The insect uses its stinger to defend its hive or nest against invaders, or to inject toxic venom into its prey to capture it. Even in small amounts, the chemicals in venom are remarkably powerful, able in some instances to paralyze prey.

Stinging insects are attracted to perfumes, bright colors, shiny objects, cosmetics, hair spray, suntan lotion, sweets, juices, soft drinks and beer. Wearing drab colors, especially green and khaki, and not wearing fragrances or scented cosmetics can help deter their attentions. There are no repellents that effectively drive away stinging insects.

sting ranges from local inflammation and hives, to swelling of the throat and breathing passages, to life-threatening, systemic anaphylaxis.

- *Mild insect-sting reactions* produce some swelling and itchy redness; these appear within 10 to 20 minutes and last a few hours before fading with no serious consequences. They may reflect local irritation, rather than an IgE-antibody reaction.

- *Moderate to serious reactions* cover an extensive local area, with a hot, boggy swelling from wrist to shoulder, for example, or from ankle to thigh, and possibly also scattered hives on the body – this is likely an IgE-mediated allergic reaction.

- *Severe, generalized allergic reactions* usually appear within seconds to minutes of an insect sting, affecting many areas of the body with itching, flushing and widespread hives and swelling of throat and tongue (which can obstruct the airway and hinder breathing); faintness, a sudden drop in blood pressure, shock, collapse and death can follow unless a life-saving epinephrine injection is given.

Warning signs of serious insect allergy

- skin-reddening in many parts of the body
- widespread itchiness, rash or hives (red welts)
- swelling of eyelids, face, hands, lips, throat
- gastric discomfort such as abdominal cramps, nausea, vomiting, diarrhea
- swelling of the tongue and larynx (voicebox), making it hard to speak or breathe
- a sense of impending doom
- rapid and/or pounding heartbeat, dizziness
- lightheadedness
- loss of consciousness, possible seizures

Diagnosing Insect Allergies

If you suspect that you have an insect allergy, get yourself med-ically assessed and properly diagnosed. Unfortunately, some people who experience even quite widespread or severe insect reactions dismiss them after the event, once the discomfort fades, without bothering to consult a physician. But anyone who has had a severe reaction should be medically evaluated, and probably allergy-tested.

Skin tests can determine the type of allergy and the insect responsible. The tests are usually postponed until about six weeks after the last insect sting, to allow IgE antibody levels to return to normal. As with other allergy tests, there may be some danger of a severe allergic reaction to venom skin tests, so the procedure should be done by a qualified allergist in a medical setting, with full emergency equipment on hand. The initial skin test solutions are much diluted, and the dose is very slowly increased, to ensure maximum safety.

Allergists would like to be able to predict who is at risk of a life-threatening insect reaction, but that's not always possi-ble. There's no reliable way to know who will have a severe allergic response before it happens. Large local reactions do *not* necessarily indicate the danger of future allergic shock; a large local swelling occurs in only 5 percent of those who later experience sting anaphylaxis. Most people who have an ana-phylactic reaction had no prior warning of it, although they must have been previously sensitized. Note, too, that people who have been stung on several occasions with no serious result may still develop a severe reaction to stings later in life.

People with other allergies such as hay fever are not neces-sarily at above-average risk of insect allergy. If one member of a family has had a severe insect reaction, other relatives won't necessarily respond in the same way. People with asthma who suffer severe insect-sting reactions are at particular risk because these may precipitate a life-threatening asthmatic attack. Also, anyone taking beta-blocker medications is at extra risk because the drug blocks the effects of epinephrine. For obvious reasons, other people at special risk are beekeepers and their families – multiple simultaneous stings can produce a massive reaction.

Deaths from Insect-Allergy Reactions

Since ancient times, writers have recorded stories of bizarre deaths from various insects as they were accidentally stepped on, swallowed or swatted, or as they attacked their unfortunate victims. The first recorded death from an insect allergy was that of King Menes, founder of the first Egyptian dynasty, who, according to the hieroglyphics on his tomb, died of a wasp sting. Another noteworthy death from a stinging insect appears in the Talmud, which tells of a holy man fatally stung while having an illicit love affair with his housekeeper. The first scientific description we have of insect allergy is a 1699 Latin account of bee-sting anaphylaxis.

No one knows exactly how many fatalities occur each year from insect stings, as some may be mistakenly attributed to other causes, such as heart attacks. Statisticians estimate that in North America 40 to 50 people die each year from insect stings, but this is likely an underestimate; many allergy-induced fatalities go unrecognized, especially if there is no record of a previous serious reaction, and if the victim was alone at the time of death. The telltale signs of anaphylaxis – the hives, flushed face and throat and tongue swelling – fade fast, leaving few clues as to the real cause of death. For every death known to be due to an insect sting, there are hundreds of near-fatal allergic reactions. But most people who die of insect-sting anaphylaxis have had no previous systemic reaction.

Fortunately, insect-sting stories are beginning to have happier endings as people become more aware of the danger and take better precautions.

Outgrowing insect allergies

Children may outgrow insect sensitivity, as illustrated in one insect-sting challenge study conducted in Germany and Austria, reported in the *Journal of Allergy and Immunology*. The study looked at 113 children, two to seventeen years old, who had suffered severe but not life-threatening insect reactions. These children were admitted to hospital and restung on their arms. This time only 13 percent had serious reactions, suggesting that the others had outgrown their insect allergy. Alternatively, these children were not really predisposed to anaphylaxis from insect stings, even though they had had a severe reaction.

For example, one Sunday afternoon when Eric, a 28-year-old rock musician, was playing in an outdoor concert, he was stung by a yellow jacket (perhaps annoyed by the noise of his electric guitar!) Within minutes Eric was covered with hives. His throat began to swell, and he began to wheeze and cough. Luckily, some bystanders recognized that his life was in danger and rushed him to the local hospital, where he was promptly treated with epinephrine.

When Eric recovered, he couldn't believe that a tiny insect could cause such a dreadful reaction. The physician suggested a course of venom injections to prevent another, possibly life-threatening episode, and referred him to a qualified allergist. He can now enjoy outdoor activities with less trepidation.

First Aid for Bites and Stings

- First, check to see if a stinger is left in the skin. Honeybees leave behind barbed stingers that can continue to pump venom into the body. Use a card or fingernail to flick off the stinger, taking care not to squeeze it in the process, as this will release more venom. Try to check what stung or bit you.
- Don't run but walk (overheating increases toxin absorption). A dip in cold water or a nearby lake (shallow water,

because of the risk of weakness and drowning) may minimize the reaction by constricting blood vessels and stimulating natural adrenalin release through the shock of
hitting cold water.

- For mild local symptoms such as redness and itching, wash
  the attack site (with antibacterial soap, if available), swab
  with antiseptic and apply ice or cold compresses to bring
  down the swelling.

- Elevate the leg, arm or other part, if possible.

- Itching may be relieved by calamine lotion, or a paste of
  baking soda and water; or you can try putting on a paste
  of commercial meat tenderizer containing papain, an
  enzyme that supposedly reduces the pain and swelling if
  used very soon after an insect sting.

- If necessary, take antihistamine tablets to reduce local
  itching. (Topical antihistamines are of uncertain benefit.)

- If itching persists, apply a steroid or combined steroid-
  antibiotic cream to reduce inflammation and prevent
  infection. Rub in the cream and cover it with plastic wrap
  secured with cellulose tape, for better absorption.

- Stay alert to the possible spread of symptoms – weakness,
  flushing and/or dizziness – and get to hospital quickly at
  the first hint of a severe reaction.

- In case of a generalized reaction, waste no time. Use epinephrine immediately, and go at once to the nearest hospital or emergency room. The epinephrine stops the
  immediate reaction, but the reaction can worsen and/or
  late reactions can occur a few hours later, so getting to
  hospital as fast as possible is a must. Even if the symptoms resolve with the injection, the person must be medically monitored. In addition to epinephrine, other
  medications, oxygen and respiratory assistance may be
  needed.

Avoiding Bites and Stings

- Have insecticide handy. Insect repellents such as diethyl-toluamide (deet) do not deter stinging insects, but will keep away mosquitoes and other biting insects. Products containing citronella oil, ethyl hexanediol and dimethyl phthalate may also repel some insects. Put repellent on the skin (avoiding the eyes) or spray it on clothes. Avoid excess repellent on children.
- Don't bother bugs and they won't bother you. Provoking an insect or panicking over it increases the chances of a sting. If a bee or wasp is in the vicinity, do not flap your arms, rush away or scream, as it may become frightened and sting in self-defense.
- If a bee or wasp comes close, remain calm and move away slowly; if it lands on you, brush it away gently. Swatting frightens insects and makes them apt to sting.
- Avoid insect attractants such as cooking smells, picnics, messy garbage, bright colors, pet food, perfumes and scented cosmetics. Don't leave uncovered food outdoors.
- Wear drab (green, tan or khaki) colors, as bright or shiny clothes attract many stinging insects (although mosquitoes like dark colors). Avoid bright colors that look like flowers and may attract bees.
- Be especially vigilant when it's humid as some insects are angrier in wet weather.
- Instruct children never to throw stones or jab sticks into insects' nests, and don't poke at insects.
- Before getting into a car, check to make sure no insects are trapped inside. If there is an insect in the car, don't swat it or try to drive off. Pull over and swish it out carefully – usually the insect will fly out if you open the window. Keep a spray can of insecticide in the vehicle to spray an errant insect.

- Be on the lookout for hidden nests – often under eaves, decks, fallen logs, compost heaps or hanging vines.
- If there are nests around the house, have an exterminator remove them. Hornets live in large paper nests; some wasps live in holes in the ground or under eaves. A local beekeeper may be willing to come to your property to relocate a bee colony.
- Locate yellow-jacket nests during the day, but wait until evening when the insects have come home to tackle them. Pour gasoline, kerosene or lye down the hole at least twice. The fumes will kill the insects – *do not light the fuel*.
- Garden cautiously. Take care not to disturb a nest of wasps, or a swarm feeding on garbage; avoid using clippers on hanging plants or places that may conceal insects or their nests. Be well covered, with long sleeves, shoes and socks.
- If a wasp or other insect is stuck in a room or against a window, trap it under a drinking glass; then slip a sheet of heavy paper between the wall and the glass and release the insect outdoors.
- Don't walk outside barefoot; wear shoes.
- Never drink from a can that has been left open outdoors. Attracted by the sweetness of the drink, insects may climb inside and give you a nasty sting on the mouth.
- If attacked by a swarm of bees or other dangerous flying insects, drop face down to the ground.
- Store garbage cans well covered and keep the area clean. Spray insecticide around the cans periodically. Be watchful when handling the garbage.
- Take care when shaking out tablecloths or towels – insects may be trapped inside.

Immunotherapy
Desensitization with venom extract can impressively reduce

the risk of severe insect allergies, providing up to 95 percent protection after a full course of injections. Over the last 20 years, immunotherapy against insect-sting allergies has improved considerably, as venom extracts have become better purified. After a course of allergy injections, even people who are highly insect-allergic can go on picnics, lie about on beaches and enjoy summers more completely, with less fear of insect attackers. "However," notes one allergist, "allergy injections are not an absolute guarantee, and someone who's had insect anaphylaxis should still carry an emergency kit – just in case."

A 1974 report of successful immunotherapy, in *The New England Journal of Medicine*, from Baltimore's Johns Hopkins University, set insect immunotherapy on the path to success. A beekeeper whose daughter had died of a bee-sting reaction was afraid for the safety of his four-year-old son, who had already suffered bee anaphylaxis. The researchers agreed to try the boy on a course of desensitizing bee-venom shots. The father was able, without ill effects, to extract venom from his worker bees for the desensitization shots. The researchers injected tiny doses of the venom into the child at intervals, gradually increasing the dose. After a two-month course, the child was challenged with a sting from a honeybee at a hospital with an emergency unit nearby, in case of disaster. He survived the challenge with only a mild reaction, and continued the venom therapy for some years. At last report, the boy (now an adult) was working alongside his father in the bee business.

A more famous example of successful immunotherapy is former U.S. president George Bush, who was stung by a bee while he was golfing in 1991. Bush, who had previously had a severe reaction to a bee sting, survived the second sting with no more than a minor welt. His survival is credited to a protective course of immunotherapy.

The U.S. allergy associations and the Canadian Society of Allergy and Clinical Immunology recommend venom injections for adults and children with IgE-mediated anaphylactic reactions to the venom of bees, hornets, wasps and yellow jackets. Children who have suffered only hives need not have the injections, since it is likely they will have similar (not worse) reactions if restung.

Venom injections (specific to the allergy-causing sting) are given weekly or twice weekly for about three months, then cut back to every six to eight weeks. The injections are continued for five years, to achieve maximum immunity. Sometimes, because of cross-reactivity, mixed venom extracts are used.

The history of venom immunotherapy

Immunotherapy against insect allergies was first tried in 1925, but up to the 1970s allergists injected the ground-up bodies of whole insects, as it was difficult to extract material from the tiny venom sacs. This seemed to work, and its popularity rose as people accidentally restung by wasps or bees lived to tell the tale, but many scientists remained skeptical.

An ingenious procedure developed in the early 1960s, now used for collecting honeybee venom, involves placing a double sheet of very thin plastic outside a beehive and covering it with a sugar-and-salt solution. As the bees descend onto the plastic, an electric current is sent through the solution, jolting them into stinging the plastic and releasing their precious tiny drops of pure bee venom.

One U.S. study divided patients into three groups: one received ground insect-body injections, another received a placebo and the third group got insect venom. The subjects were then challenged by being restung. Sixty percent of those given whole-body extracts or the placebo suffered severe reactions, while only one person (5 percent) given pure venom shots suffered a reaction.

If whole insect-body injections were no better than a placebo, why had whole-body treatment survived so long? Perhaps because many people with venom reactions naturally lose their insect sensitivity over time. Subsequent studies have established that 95 percent of those who receive pure, specific venom immunotherapy develop long-term tolerance to that type of insect. Pure insect venoms are now the preferred therapy.

As a generalized allergic reaction occurs in about 10 percent of people given venom-extract desensitization, immunotherapy should be undertaken only by trained, certified allergists in a place with full emergency backup. Those on beta-blocking drugs (for high blood pressure or other ailments) are at increased risk of serious reactions and should not be offered immunotherapy while taking these medications.

Occasionally, in special situations, allergy injections are given on a speeded-up schedule, with increasing venom doses being given over a few hours or days, and periodic booster shots thereafter. In one case, a 13-year-old boy who had suffered a severe sting reaction several years earlier wished to go tree planting in Northern Ontario. As he had a high likelihood of being restung up north, the boy was given a "rush session" of venom shots in hospital. Over a three-day period he received approximately hourly injections of venom, until he could tolerate the equivalent of about two stings. Thus desensitized, he set off to the bush with fewer worries.

Sorting Out the Biters

Black flies, horseflies, deerflies, bedbugs, midges, lice, fleas, mosquitoes and most ants cause mainly local reactions. Enzymes in their salivary secretions soften human skin and dilate the blood vessels, causing itchiness, redness and inflammation. Discomfort can stem from direct toxic irritation, rather than an immune-system reaction. Rubbing or scratching the site can spread the swelling and infect the area. Although systemic reactions are rare, isolated cases of death from anaphylaxis – mostly due to black fly, mosquito and deerfly bites – have been reported.

Fire ants – accidentally shipped into the U.S. from Uruguay and Argentina in sod and agricultural products at the turn of the century – have since migrated north. They are now widespread across the southern U.S. from Florida to Mississippi, Oklahoma and Texas. Similar but less cold-sensitive ants have reportedly advanced as far north as New Jersey but have not so far made it to Canada. The fire ant's attack is ferocious; 85,000 Americans seek medical attention each year for their burning, painful bites. In urban U.S. areas infested with fire ants, it is estimated that 30 to 60 percent of residents are bitten every year, about 1 percent suffering anaphylaxis. Some deaths have been reported. Fire ants live in mounds, with as many as 200 colonies per acre.

Fire Ant

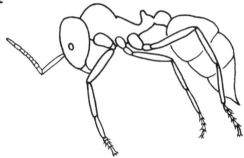

Sorting Out the Stingers

Honeybees, with squat, hairy bodies and yellow and black markings, live in hives in old trees, rock crevices or corners of houses and sheds. From spring to late September they gather nectar from flowers. *Bumblebees* are larger than honeybees, with darker markings, and nest in holes in trees. Honeybees and bumblebees are relatively docile, unlikely to sting unless provoked. The stinger is a tiny sharp needle with backwards-pointing barbs, which stays lodged in the skin after a sting. Bees can sting only once, after which they die.

African killer bees were bred in Brazil in the 1950s by cross-ing an imported African bee with a Brazilian species to produce more honey. The new breed escaped and moved north, reaching Mexico and the southern U.S. (Arizona, Texas, California) by the 1990s. These bees are very aggressive, and the slightest disturbance may provoke them to a frenzy and unprovoked attack, although their venom is no more allergenic or lethal than that of the gentler honeybee.

Bee

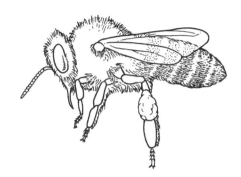

Yellow-faced and white-faced hornets nest in trees and shrubs and under house eaves. Although their gray, paper-like nests are small, they are usually visible. White-faced and bald-faced hornets have large, thick bodies and live in round nests in trees.

Wasps are easily distinguished by their slender, pinched waists. They nest under eaves and rafters. When the weather

Wasp and Hornet

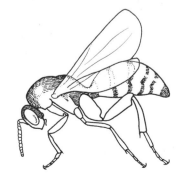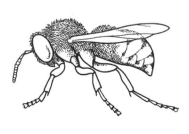

turns cold some seek a haven indoors, so be on the lookout for sleepy wasps nestled in attics or corners. Wasps and hornets are known for their aggressive character – hence our expressions "waspish" and "stirring up a hornets' nest." They may sting repeatedly even if not provoked, and do not leave behind a stinger.

Yellow jackets have slim, elongated bodies with black and yellow markings; they live in holes in the ground, or under logs or rocks, and are easily disturbed by gardening or lawn mowing. They like to eat sweets, are often found near rotten fruit and garbage and are drawn to bright colors. Like wasps and hornets, they sting even if unprovoked and leave behind no stinger, so they can attack repeatedly.

Yellow Jacket

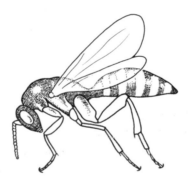

T W E L V E

Skin Allergies

Many people have an occasional skin rash that goes away on its own before any cause is found. Some rashes, however, arise from allergic conditions, including urticaria (hives), contact dermatitis and atopic dermatitis (regarded as an allergic reaction although the triggers may not be known). None of these is contagious; they are due to personal immune-system changes, and are not spread person to person.

Hives are itchy, white, raised weals surrounded by red inflamed areas or pink blotches. They can be sudden and acute, or chronic and long-lasting.

Atopic dermatitis – commonly called *eczema* – is primarily a childhood disorder, consisting of a red, itchy skin rash with rough, flaky or wet, oozy patches.

Contact dermatitis is a skin rash that can be allergic or irritant in nature.

URTICARIA (HIVES)

Hives are usually due to an allergic trigger that stimulates mast cells in the skin to release histamine (and other mediators), making blood vessels dilate and become "leaky," leading to inflammation and swelling. The skin lesion or "hive" – a roundish, red lump with a clearly demarcated border and possibly a paler center – may look like a mosquito bite or a large, raised welt. Hives range from pinhead-sized lesions to swellings over 12 inches (30 cm) across. They can appear anywhere on the body, and are sometimes scattered over one or two areas. In severe cases the whole face and body may be covered with inflamed, itchy skin bumps or blotches. The eruption may be accompanied by *angioedema* – swelling of deeper skin layers, often in the face, tongue, hands or feet, with a painful, burning sensation. If angioedema makes the throat or larynx swell severely, it impedes breathing and can be a life-threatening emergency, requiring immediate epinephrine injection.

In diagnosing and managing hives, physicians first determine whether the condition is "acute" or "chronic" – that is, persisting for six weeks or more. Hives can be sporadic, coming and going unpredictably. Although each individual hive clears within 24 to 48 hours, new lesions can appear, so attacks can linger. But acute episodes usually clear within a few days to a week, leaving no trace. Chronic cases may persist for months to years.

There are no good statistics on the number of people suffering from hives, as those with mild or transient attacks may not seek medical advice. Surveys suggest that as much as 15 to 20 percent of the North American population has an occasional bout of acute hives, most often as adults. Attacks are often triggered by a food, drug, infection, insect bite or other allergen.

In about 15 percent of people with hives, a physical factor such as pressure, extremes of heat or cold, sunlight or even exercise triggers the skin eruption.

Hives can arise from

an allergy to:
- medications (such as penicillin, ASA, sulfonamides)
- insect stings
- airborne allergens (such as pollens – a rare cause)
- certain foods

an allergy-like reaction to:
- drugs such as opiates, salicylates (e.g., ASA/aspirin), NSAIDs and other substances that cause direct histamine release
- food additives (e.g., tartrazine)
- radiocontrast media (used for X-rays)
- insect bites (bedbugs, fleas, mosquitoes)

physical causes:
- dermatographism (skin easily irritated by pressure or slight trauma such as pressure from tight clothing, e.g., belts)
- exposure to heat or cold
- sunlight
- exercise or stress

specific disorders:
- connective tissue disorders (for example, lupus erythematosus, Sjögren's syndrome)
- hyperthyroidism (thyroid overactivity)
- lymphomas (cancers of the lymph glands)
- infections (e.g., viral hepatitis, mononucleosis)

Distinguishing Acute and Chronic Hives

Urticaria is classified as "acute" or "chronic" depending on its duration. *Acute urticaria* is an attack of hives that lasts less than six weeks (usually just a few days). It's usually triggered by a food, insect or drug but may accompany an infection, such as a common cold or strep throat, hepatitis, mononucleosis and some fungal and parasitic infections; it can also be provoked by a blood transfusion. Often, the trigger is not found. Penicillin and a few other drugs are among the most common causes of short-lasting, acute hives. Occasionally, the hives persist for a week or so after people stop taking the drug. Hives that occur along with other allergic reactions usually fade within hours to days, as the immune response vanishes, and generally respond well to antihistamines, not reappearing unless there's a further encounter with the triggering agent.

In a typical case, someone takes a medication to which he or she is allergic, and within minutes itchy red weals appear on the face or other parts of the body. For example, by the time he was two years old Byron had had many ear infections, which were usually treated with antibiotics, often penicillin. Then he suddenly developed generalized hives while he was on the penicillin. The hives cleared up with antihistamines. Later, a skin prick test found that Byron was allergic to penicillin, but not to any other substances tried. Byron's parents had to make sure the child was never again given penicillin, as the next reaction could be more severe. To warn health professionals who may treat him, Byron wears a medical-alert bracelet listing his penicillin allergy.

"In many cases of acute hives," notes one expert, "no triggering cause can be traced." Being a self-limiting disorder, acute hives may need no treatment other than antihistamines and, rarely, a short burst of corticosteroid therapy.

Chronic urticaria is an attack of hives that lasts longer than six weeks. It can settle into a persistent disorder lasting for months to years, flaring every day or several times a week – a condition that's hard to eradicate, as its causes are often impossible to determine. But regardless of its origins, the hiving process can be controlled or dampened by the use of antihistamines.

Chronic urticaria rarely results from an IgE-mediated allergy, but may arise from a delayed type IV immunological response (see Chapter Two). About 15 to 20 percent of people with chronic hives also have physical urticaria (see below). In a small group of those with chronic hives the problem stems from an infection, immune-system disease or other identifiable disorder. Some cases are thought to be related to autoimmune reactions due to antibodies that attack the body's own tissues. Heredity plays a role, as some forms tend to run in families.

Tracking the origins of chronic hives can challenge the best of allergists. Tests often fail to uncover any trigger, and in the overwhelming majority of cases no reason is ever found; the hives are simply designated "of no known cause." The condition can be most distressing to those afflicted, and their caregivers – especially if, despite much time and effort spent pursuing every conceivable avenue, no cause can be determined.

Quite often, a person plagued by hives is convinced that a certain food (or food additive) – say, shrimp, eggs or a food dye – is to blame, and may coerce the allergist into doing exhaustive tests to confirm the suspicion, only to find that no dietary ingredient provokes the skin eruption. Sometimes an elimination diet is tried – perhaps cutting out all foods except, say, rice and lamb, adding items back one by one to see if the hives reappear – yet the search still ends in failure.

"There's no use doing batteries of exhaustive, time-consuming and anxiety-provoking medical investigations and tests in most cases," observes one University of Toronto immunologist, "because, likely as not, one ends up not finding the cause of chronic urticaria. The reason often remains elusive and for the vast majority – 80 to 85 percent – no cause is ever found. In many cases, people must learn to live with the condition and relieve symptoms with whatever works best for them."

Managing Acute and Chronic Hives

The treatment of urticaria depends first and foremost on taking a careful history, trying to identify any causes and then avoiding or removing them. While a minor bout of hives will probably disappear on its own, if hives persist for days, or recur, a physician should always be consulted.

Antihistamines are the first line of treatment. For most people, the first-generation antihistamines are all that's needed. Hydroxyzine has been found most effective, and other useful antihistamines include chlorpheniramine and diphenhydramine. Of the second-generation antihistamines, cetirizine, which also has some anti-inflammatory action, may be especially useful. If the usual H_1-blocking antihistamines don't work, a physician may prescribe histamine H_2 blockers such as cimetidine (Tagamet), ranitidine (Zantac) or famotidine (Pepcid). (See Chapter Five for more about antihistamines.) Primarily stomach-ulcer drugs, these act on histamine receptors in the large blood vessels and gut, and also affect the immune system in ways that may relieve hives. You may have to try several medications before you find the right combination. Should none of the usual approaches bring relief, a short course of oral corticosteroids (for a week or so) may be suggested. Above all, sufferers need plenty of support for what can be a very upsetting disorder.

People with hives should avoid common irritants such as wool clothing next to the skin, detergents, perfumes and soaps, and are advised not to take medications containing ASA, as these compounds trigger the release of histamine and can aggravate hives.

Note: *If you have severe hives with extensive swelling (perhaps breathing difficulties), get to a hospital emergency department at once. It could be the preliminary stage of anaphylactic shock.*

Physical Urticaria

Cold urticaria (cold-triggered hives) occurs suddenly from a cold wind, immersion in very cold water or an ice-cube applied to the skin. Your lips may swell after you eat ice cream, or your hands may swell after you hold a cold object or immerse them in icy water. (The effects may be worst on rewarming.) Total body exposure – such as diving into a cold lake – can trigger a massive histamine release, causing anaphylaxis, with the risk of sudden death. Wear protective clothing in cold weather, and be cautious about swimming in cold water – and always try to swim with a buddy. The condition can appear and disappear spontaneously or can last a lifetime; it may have a genetic component, as some forms run in families. Therapy is with antihistamines; the drug cyproheptadine is especially helpful.

Cholinergic urticaria (heat-triggered hives) can be local (occurring in small areas of the skin exposed to heat), but is usually generalized. Small hives often first appear on the neck and upper body, then spread all over, perhaps with considerable swelling. The condition can be triggered by any heat – a very hot shower, intense exercise or a fever. The problem is most common in teens and young adults. Hydroxyzine is the drug of choice, being more effective than other antihistamines for this condition.

Delayed pressure urticaria, with deep, painful hives and swelling arising from gradual pressure – for example, carrying a heavy knapsack or bag on the shoulders for a few hours, or wearing a tight belt or watch strap – affects about 11 percent of those with chronic hives. Along with the hives, some people have flu-like symptoms and joint pains.

Solar urticaria – triggered by exposure to the sun's ultraviolet rays, and also other forms of light – is a rare form of very itchy hives that usually fades within a few hours.

Dermatographism – a curious form of urticaria – literally means "write on the skin," because slight pressure can actually sign a name across the person's back. The red welts develop in response to slight rubbing, friction or even firm stroking. The condition affects 36 percent of all those who suffer from physical urticaria, and 2 percent of the North American population at large. It is easily diagnosed by stroking the skin and observing the white line that appears within minutes and soon turns red and itchy. Some people describe a "skin crawling" sensation. Antihistamines, especially diphenhydramine, can relieve the discomfort.

Exercise-induced hives is a condition where vigorous exercise produces severe hives (sometimes huge weals), along with swelling, wheezing, a drop in blood pressure and other symptoms of allergic shock or anaphylaxis. It's quite often seen in athletes. But although it's similar to heat-induced urticaria, it can be distinguished from it because the hives don't appear on exposure to heat alone (such as a hot shower), but only with exercise. People with exercise-induced hives often have other allergies, including other forms of physical urticaria. Sometimes the exercise-induced allergy is linked to eating a meal shortly beforehand, or to the consumption of specific foods (such as shellfish or celery) before exercise. (See also Chapter 10.)

ATOPIC DERMATITIS

Atopic (allergic) dermatitis is especially common in young children. The term "eczema" – which means "boiling over" – is popularly used by the public (and even by some health professionals) to mean the infantile form of atopic dermatitis, but modern dermatologists use the word to describe the inflamed, crusting skin eruption that also occurs in other disorders such as scabies (a mite infection), athlete's foot and seborrheic dermatitis (a greasy, yellowish skin condition on the scalp, nasal folds and elsewhere). "Dermatitis" is an all-inclusive term for an inflamed skin rash.

Many different terms have been used to describe atopic dermatitis; one reviewer in the 1970s found 20 different synonyms for this skin condition. We will use the term "atopic dermatitis" to describe a specific allergy-related skin condition characterized by eczema-like, scaling, weepy skin lesions.

Atopic dermatitis is an inherited, chronic condition. Although it can affect people of any age, in the Western world it afflicts primarily young children, and can start up in infants almost from birth on. It often appears within the first year of life – commonly within the first three months – surfacing by age two in 95 percent of cases. It was first described in Europe during the late 1800s, as "Besnier's prurigo." Many of those affected come from allergy-prone families. About one-third of children with atopic dermatitis develop asthma, and about 25 percent later suffer from hay fever or other inhalant allergies.

Atopic dermatitis ranges from mild to disablingly severe, with eczema-like skin eruptions that are moist and weepy or dry and scaly with cracked and roughened skin, and sometimes even appears as pebbly *ichthyosis* ("fish skin"). The disease has flare-ups and periods of remission. During a flare-up there can be considerable swelling and inflammation. In its smoldering or "subacute" form, affected areas are just dry, rough patches. In older children, the skin can become "lichenified" (thickened, like lichen), with deepened or furrowed lines, especially on the limbs. The more severe the condition, the likelier it is to be long-lasting.

Areas of atopic dermatitis easily become infected with bacteria such as *Staphylococcus aureus*, and viruses such as *Herpes simplex*, making the condition flare. The famous "boils of Job" are said by some medical historians to have been badly infected eczema.

Although its causes remain unknown, atopic dermatitis is now viewed primarily as a genetically based skin disorder involving IgE antibody overproduction, activation of mast cells, a predisposition to *xerosis* (dry skin), and abnormal turnover of epidermal (outer-layer) skin. If there's a family history of the condition – if either or both parents have or had atopic dermatitis – there's a high likelihood that the children will also be affected, although the exact way it's inherited isn't yet clear.

Who Gets Atopic Dermatitis?

Although its precise incidence is hard to assess, as those with mild eczema may not seek medical attention, there seems to have been a marked rise in atopic dermatitis in Western countries over the last 30 years. (The apparent increase may reflect improved diagnosis.) Currently, in North America and Europe, an estimated 10 to 15 percent of infants under one year old have some degree of atopic dermatitis, as well as 5 percent of schoolchildren and about 2 percent of adults. In over 60 percent of cases, there's a family history of allergic disorders. The incidence is lower in developing countries. Atopic dermatitis affects all races, but is particularly common in Caucasian and Chinese people, especially in industrialized countries. Although both sexes are equally susceptible in infancy, more adult women than men have it. Some studies suggest that the disorder is particularly prevalent among the children of recent immigrants to industrialized countries such as the U.S. and Canada.

Infants frequently outgrow eczema, and by the time they are toddlers the disorder has gone in many cases. By adolescence half the affected infants have outgrown this skin affliction, and it clears in 90 percent of cases by age 20. However, for children and teens the condition can have a devastating impact, profoundly disrupting family, social, school and work life.

Eczema Varies through Childhood

In the infant form (from birth to age two), the eczema appears as scaly crusted patches or a weepy rash, typically on the face – on the cheeks and chin – and on the sides of the arms and lower legs. The infant's scalp and hair may be dry, itchy and scaling. The diaper area is often spared, possibly because it stays moist and prevents the skin dryness typical of eczema. Atopic dermatitis during infancy can herald an allergic predisposition, with other allergies to follow, even years after the eczema has vanished.

The childhood form, seen from age two through to puberty, appears as scaly patches that often become rough and pebbled – most often behind the knees, inside the elbows, at the wrists, ankles, buttock creases, behind the ears and in the neck folds. It worsens in areas that get sweaty. In the neck folds, the red patches may become rippled and brown – a hallmark of atopic dermatitis. Eczematous children often have buffed, shiny fingernails from the perpetual rubbing. Further telltale features are the exaggeratedly furrowed skin markings, or "hyperlinearity," on the palms of the hands and soles of the feet. Hypopigmented (depigmented) patches may be scattered on the face or body – these are especially noticeable in black-skinned people. The "Dennie-Morgan" fold beneath the eyes is almost diagnostic of the disorder. The eyes may also be itchy and red with a painful eye inflammation called "vernal conjunctivitis." (See Chapter Thirteen.)

Childhood atopic dermatitis may continue into adolescence, flaring from time to time, plaguing teens with a scaly rash in areas similar to those of childhood (behind the knees, on elbows and wrists), and also around the eyelids and nipples and sometimes in the groin. However, even severely crusted eczema rarely leaves lasting scars, unless it becomes infected. Sometimes, childhood eczema will disappear only to reappear in adulthood. Adult forms are diffusely scattered, but often occur around the eyes and mouth.

Diagnosing Atopic Dermatitis

The clues to diagnosing atopic dermatitis are the dry, roughened, intensely itchy eczema, endless scratching and a family history of allergies. To confirm the diagnosis, other conditions that cause eczema such as scabies, seborrheic dermatitis, fungal infections, immunodeficiency and contact dermatitis must be excluded.

In taking a history, the physician will ask about scratching, sleep disturbance, possible aggravating factors, allergies in the family, diet, and the disorder's effects on school, social life, career and emotional state. The physician looks for signs of bacterial infection (crusting, pus or oozing) and herpes infection. Allergy skin tests may be considered but are of little diagnostic value. If the eczema responds well to treatment with topical corticosteroids, no further diagnostic tests are necessary.

Itchiness Is the Hallmark

Itchiness is the most characteristic and bothersome feature of atopic dermatitis – sometimes bad enough to disturb sleep, make infants claw at their skin and rub against any available object – a pillow or the sides of the cot – trying to relieve the sometimes unbearable itch. The child's scratching can drive parents and other caretakers berserk in their efforts to stop the baby from rubbing its skin raw.

Some physicians believe it's not so much the skin lesions but the fierce scratching that produces the crusted sores and thickened skin. As the French dermatologist Jacquet said of the condition at the turn of the century, "It is not the rash that itches, but the itch that rashes." The paradox was well illustrated by a 1936 experiment at Washington University. A two-year-old child with severe eczema triggered by wheat was treated in hospital until his skin cleared. Half the child's body was then wrapped in bandages, the rest left unbandaged, and the child was fed wheat crackers. His skin began to itch and after a whole night's scratching his exposed skin was torn, raw and eczematous, but the skin under the bandages remained unblemished and clear of any rash.

However, experts point out that the skin eruption may appear in very young infants, at around three months of age, before the "itch–scratch" mechanism develops.

Causes and Predisposing Factors

Atopic dermatitis is a complex disorder with no clear-cut causes. "Despite the unknown origin of the disease," says one dermatologist, "newer findings and theories add to the already existing confusion, and none of the explanations offered clarifies the underlying mechanism of atopic dermatitis. The basic defect remains a mystery."

However, there are some known predisposing factors:

- *Genetic background.* The condition tends to run in families, sometimes together with asthma and hay fever. One of the first atopic families described may be that of the Emperor Augustus. According to his biographer Sartorius, the Roman emperor suffered from an itchy skin disease that may have been atopic dermatitis. He also had hay fever and tightness of the chest, which could have been asthma. The grandson of Augustus, the Emperor Claudius, also suffered from hay fever and his great-grandnephew Britannicus is supposed to have had what we would call a horse allergy.

- *Immunological abnormalities.* These may include defects in white blood cells, and delayed hypersensitivity reactions (involving T-cells). IgE-antibody levels are elevated in about 80 percent of children with atopic dermatitis, although their exact role is not understood.

- *Skin abnormalities.* People prone to atopic dermatitis often have skin that differs biochemically from normal skin and is much drier, with decreased water-binding capacity. Their skin may be extra-sensitive to irritants such as chafing clothes, neck tags or rough seams. Easily irritated skin can develop eczema from sweating, or from changes in humidity or temperature, and the condition may flare in dry conditions or if the skin is exposed to soaps, fragrances or hot water.

What Role Do Dust Mites and Food Allergens Play?

Inhaled allergens such as dust-mite feces are increasingly suspected of inducing atopic dermatitis. One recent study found that dust control reduced the severity of the disorder. And in a Japanese study of "clean room" therapy, 30 people with severe eczema who had demonstrable dust-mite sensitivity found their skin condition cleared up when they were kept in houses free of dust mites, or in dust-free hospital rooms. But most allergists are skeptical about the role of dust mites in this condition, and do not suggest rigorous mite-removing efforts or scrupulous dust-control measures. There is little proof that dust-mite elimination will be beneficial – but if you suspect it might, vacuum well, avoid wall-to-wall carpeting, cover mattresses and pillows with impermeable covers and wash bedding once weekly in very hot water. Atopic dermatitis often flares during the pollen season.

Various foods have also come under suspicion as triggers, and many parents of infants and toddlers with atopic dermatitis blame the disorder on a food allergy. Some even think that several foods worsen their child's condition, though children very rarely react to more than one food. A few studies have linked worsening eczema to certain foods. In a 1985 double-blind study reported in the *Journal of Pediatrics*, more than half of 113 infants with severe atopic dermatitis had a skin reaction when they were fed certain foods such as eggs, milk, peanut, fish, soy or wheat. When taken off these foods, some, though not all, showed considerable skin improvement. Overall, the evidence shows that less than 10 percent of childhood atopic dermatitis can be traced in any way to a food allergy, and then mainly in severe cases.

For example, Alison's mother was worried about her four-month-old baby's itchy rash, which started on her cheeks and chin, spreading to the lower legs and arms. Alison was constantly rubbing and scratching the rash, only making it worse. She was irritable, fussy and clearly in distress. Convinced that her daughter was allergic to something, Alison's mother took her to the pediatrician. A careful history established that the child's mother had asthma and her older sister suffered from hay fever. The physician prescribed a corticosteroid cream with careful bathing instructions, which Alison's mother meticulously followed. The rash cleared within a few days.

Alison is a textbook case of infantile eczema, experiencing her first bout in early infancy. According to one estimate, 90 percent of atopic dermatitis begins before age five, and most of that before age two. Alison's itchy eczema occurred in the classic infantile pattern – on the face, particularly the cheeks and chin. Like Alison, many with eczema come from allergy-prone families. Alison's eczema is fairly severe, which may mean it will persist longer than usual. Her condition responded well to the topical steroid cream, but it soon came back.

"Although parents often demand food tests, and allergists

may comply," notes one dermatologist at a Toronto children's hospital, "skin and blood tests do *not* accurately diagnose food-induced eczema. Eating a food that skin-tests positive does *not* necessarily worsen the eczema." The tests create confusion because a positive result may convince parents that their child's eczema comes from certain foods. But most allergists believe foods have been unjustly blamed for causing atopic dermatitis, leading to sometimes health-endangering dietary restriction. Unfortunately, skin tests are notoriously inaccurate in pinpointing a food as the cause of atopic dermatitis, so there is no easy way to prove or disprove the connection.

Managing Atopic Dermatitis

Although there's no cure, eczema can be controlled. Meticulously regular application of moisturizers is essential to replenish and retain water in the skin. Avoidance of irritants such as harsh soaps and rough clothing is an integral part of treatment. Antibiotics may be needed to treat any infection present.

Topical corticosteroid ointments are the mainstay of treatment to reduce the inflammation, stop itching and reduce scratching. Mild preparations are used on the face, stronger ones on the rest of the body.

Special skin care is essential. Mild, unscented soaps are a must. After bathing (perhaps with a capful of oil in the bathwater), the skin should be left wet and moisturizer applied to the damp skin at once. Since eczematous skin is dry, it must be regularly lubricated with after-bath emollients.

Other possible therapies include use of ultraviolet (UVB) light, although its benefits fade when therapy stops. Oral antihistamines may help, but their main benefit seems to be a sedating effect that helps distressed children sleep at night. In general, therapy allows those affected to carry on a normal life with minimal disruption, although some cases are stubbornly resistant.

Topical Corticosteroid Therapy: Safe and Effective

For greatest effectiveness, corticosteroid ointments free of sensitizers are used for eczema, except in hairy or very moist areas where less greasy creams may be better. Creams are best for the scalp. For the face, eyelids, groin and armpits a low-potency steroid is advised; check labels carefully to see which product is meant for which part of the body.

For mild eczema, a low-dose (1 percent) hydrocortisone product will usually clear up the problem.

For more severe cases – or if the rash affects thicker skin (as on the hands and feet) or the lesions are crusty, in which case steroids are less easily absorbed – stronger forms such as betamethasone valerate or triamcinolone may be prescribed. Oral corticosteroids are a "last resort" and are rarely warranted, especially as there can be a rebound flare of eczema when they're stopped.

Many parents are afraid of using even topical corticosteroids for their children; British surveys find that one reason treatment fails is that people fear side-effects of steroid medications and so don't use enough. However, used correctly at the right dosages, these medications are safe and effective, and there are few side-effects from the use of topical corticosteroids in children. Ask your physician to explain the side-effects, and to indicate precisely how much ointment should be applied, when and where.

A few cautions about corticosteroid use:

- Use low-dose (1 percent) hydrocortisone on the face and delicate areas such as the groin. Prolonged use of stronger

---

Remedies for atopic dermatitis

Low-potency steroids
- hydrocortisone (1 percent or less) – some available over the counter
- desonide

Medium-potency steroids
- triamcinolone – 0.0 to 0.1 percent
- betamethasone – 0.05 to 0.1 percent, ointment or cream.

Super-potency steroids
- Diprolene (betamethasone) – 0.25 percent cream, ointment or lotion

Other medications
- tar ointments: a former eczema remedy, still sometimes used, often in combination with a mild topical corticosteroid. They may be an excellent treatment for eczema but have a slight odor, so are best used at night. Today's products are less staining than those of the past
- antihistamines: of uncertain benefit, but may help relieve the itch and promote sleep. Ketotifen is a useful itch-reliever. Sedating antihistamines such as diphenhydramine may be worth a try when itching keeps children up at night, especially as much of the skin damage from scratching happens at night. The newer, nonsedating antihistamines are not effective for this condition
- acyclovir for herpes viruses, and antibiotics against bacteria, are helpful. A few experts suggest that long-term antibiotic therapy may help prevent recurrences, but others oppose prolonged antibiotics because of the risk of drug-resistant bacterial strains
- new medications for severe atopic dermatitis, including cyclosporin, an immunosuppressant with some promise for adults

---

corticosteroids can cause skin thinning and spider capillaries (very fine, visible blood vessels).
- For best penetration, apply corticosteroids on moist skin right after bathing.
- Prolonged use of all topical steroid preparations requires medical supervision.

Special Bathing Care for Atopic Dermatitis
Recommendations for bathing are somewhat divergent, with

different specialists offering different advice. In years past, sufferers were told to bathe infrequently in order not to dry out the skin. Nowadays, most dermatologists encourage frequent bathing – at least once daily, sometimes more – provided moisturizers are lavishly applied immediately afterwards to trap water in the skin.

Besides regular tub baths (better than showers, which are more drying), some dermatologists suggest adding oatmeal to the water to soothe the skin, and unscented bath oils – though these may be a hazard, owing to the risk of slipping. Most suggest that the skin be left wet after bathing, and that non-inflamed areas be lubricated at once with moisturizing emollients, immediately on exiting the tub.

The choice of moisturizing product can be discussed with your healthcare provider. In general, emollients or ointments are most effective, but creams can replace them in humid conditions. Lotions often contain alcohol and can be both drying and irritating; they are also higher in water content, so they are less effective moisturizers than emollients or creams. Thickened, pebbly areas are poorly penetrated by creams and need a rich emollient or ointment such as petrolatum.

Bathing tips
- The right tub-soaking time is much debated, but many dermatologists suggest five to ten minutes.
- Do not make the bathwater too hot, as hot water releases histamine; most suggest tepid water.
- Make bathtime fun for young children with water toys; older children might listen to a tape or read while soaking.
- Use the least amount of soap possible, and choose mild brands; avoid bubble bath.
- After the bath, apply medication and moisturize at once.

Moisturizing tips
- Use moisturizer liberally and frequently.
- Apply moisturizing emollient lavishly to damp skin. (Without moisturizers the water evaporates, leaving the skin drier than before.)
- Choose the moisturizer that's best for your skin. In general, the oilier the product, the more effective it is, emollients (ointments) being better moisturizers than creams or lotions. Cheap (but greasy) petrolatum is very effective; less greasy products include Lubriderm, Keri lotion and Nutraderm cream. Adolescents in particular may shun greasy products and need advice in choosing the right moisturizer.

Other useful things to do
- Keep the temperature of the house (or at least the bedrooms) low and the humidity high.
- Protect skin from dry weather with creams and emollients before going outdoors and at bedtime.
- Keep fingernails short and clean so there is less chance of tearing and infecting the skin. Children may have to wear gloves at night.
- Wear 100 percent cotton next to the skin all year round, as it is less likely to irritate it than wool, silk, polyester or nylon.
- Use only mild detergent for washing clothes. Rinse clothes several times; many detergents are irritating. Avoid bleach and fabric softeners.
- When eczema flares, apply corticosteroid ointment three times a day, or as prescribed.
- Avoid situations that increase sweating – overheated places, tight clothing, heavy bedding.
- Try to keep cool: take children to wading pools in hot

weather; during summer months, air-condition your home if possible.

- Use a barrier petrolatum or other emollient before entering a chlorinated pool.
- Avoid strolls through grass at pollination time, which can aggravate the skin irritation.

Coping with Difficult Eczema

Most atopic dermatitis will clear with mild corticosteroid therapy, but for some people the skin condition is chronic, difficult and frustrating to treat. Surveys show that many people find the disorder seriously disrupts their everyday lives. The British Association of Dermatologists and the Royal College of Physicians in London published guidelines in 1995 to help those coping with difficult eczema. They emphasized the many preventable treatment failures – in particular, blaming the fact that people are poorly informed about the condition. They suggested asking a dermatologist or allergist for clear instructions about medications, bathing, moisturizers and other details, and discussing worries about medication side-effects. Request written instructions, or write things down yourself, and watch for infections – oozing patches with pus – which need prompt attention.

Some reasons for treatment failure

- not following instructions, or not taking medication
- corticosteroid medication not strong enough
- too little moisturizer applied too infrequently
- bacterial or viral infection that exacerbates the eczema not being promptly treated with antibiotics
- repeated exposure to irritants such as perfumes
- rubbing because of the persistent itch, developing secondary infection
- not doing everything possible – whatever works – to control the itchiness and avoid scratching

Managing Atopic Dermatitis Can Be Stressful

Some children afflicted by atopic dermatitis are painfully aware of their blemished skin, and embarrassed by it. They may be taunted by schoolmates and siblings and suffer acute emotional distress. Caring for a child with eczema can be physically and mentally exhausting, with sleepless nights, and with creative abilities stretched to capacity to stop the scratching, and added guilt feelings. Experts emphasize that although stress does not cause atopic dermatitis, the condition is stressful to manage, often has considerable psychological effect and can upset family dynamics. Uncomfortable, itchy children who need vigilance and frequent skin care tend to become manipulative. They quickly realize that their parents will do anything to avoid stress-producing discipline. A firm, direct approach is usually advised, with diversionary tactics when scratching is likely to be worst, to keep the child's hands occupied. Parents may benefit from counseling on ways to manage the situation.

CONTACT DERMATITIS

There are two main types of contact dermatitis:

- *irritant* contact dermatitis, which is *non-allergic* and results from an irritating substance that touches the skin and causes a rash, perhaps with blisters;
- *allergic* contact dermatitis, due to an allergen touching the skin. This is usually a delayed type IV allergy. One familiar example of allergic contact dermatitis is poison ivy rash, with its red blisters appearing in the area of contact within 12 to 48 hours of a sensitized person being exposed to the plant. With simple sleuthing you can often trace the cause of allergic contact dermatitis, perhaps by backtracking over your activities or listing new personal products you've tried. (Also note new supplies of your old

favorites, as manufacturers may change product formulas without saying so on the label.)

Most dermatitis is due to irritants, not allergens. For instance, battery acid will cause a strong inflammatory reaction in anyone; reddened "dishpan hands" can result from soaking in hot water or washing with drying soaps. But some substances can be both irritant and allergenic; the irritation makes it easier for allergens to get into the skin.

Contact Allergens Are Everywhere

At last count, some 2,800 different substances were being blamed for contact allergies; with new products flooding the market, contact dermatitis is an ever-expanding problem. People get *latex allergy* from wearing surgical gloves; *consort dermatitis* from products worn by a partner, such as cologne or condoms; *fiddler's fingers*, a rash on the hands, from violin rosin. Workers become allergic to cement, flour and other substances encountered on the job, and innumerable household and personal-care products can cause a reaction. Fortunately, the vast majority of these allergies are not serious, and the contact allergen is often easy to identify and avoid. For example, one of the most common triggers of allergic contact dermatitis – nickel – is often used in body jewelry; be sure you know what you're buying.

Although an occasional skin rash may not be too bothersome, contact dermatitis can be a distressing, even disabling disorder. Occupational contact dermatitis can make life miserable for industrial workers.

Contact can occur via several routes:
- *occasional skin contact* – for example, with hair dye, bubble bath, perfume or detergent
- *airborne contact*, as with fragrances; one woman devel-

oped a contact reaction when she was accidentally sprayed
with perfume during a department-store demonstration
- *ingestion of food or drink,* for example, consuming a dye
  or nickel in food. A low-nickel diet may clear up nickel-
  induced dermatitis.
- *photocontact,* through a chemical in conjunction with
  ultraviolet light. Someone who sprays on a fragrance and
  then goes into the sunlight may break out in red blotches
  (which become brown) precisely where the perfume was
  applied. Musk ambrette, an ingredient popular in 1970s
  aftershave, was a common cause of photocontact dermatitis. Some medications, such as erythromycin, are
  notorious for causing allergic photocontact dermatitis.

How Common Is Contact Dermatitis?

There are few statistics on the number of people who suffer
from allergic contact dermatitis, partly because people with
minor skin problems often don't seek medical care. Nor is
there any "gold standard" for diagnosing the condition, so
surveys are difficult to carry out. However, surveys in Ontario
estimate that contact dermatitis accounts for about 25 percent
of all worker-compensation health claims. Certain occupa-
tions pose greater risks than others. The chromium often
found in cement is a highly sensitizing substance, and 50
percent of cement workers in North America are allergic to
it. Chromium is so sensitizing that its use in cement has been
banned in certain places such as Singapore. Allergic dermatitis is also a common problem for auto manufacturing employees exposed to highly sensitizing cutting oils, used as metal
coolants. Others at risk of allergic contact dermatitis are those
employed in the leather, printing, dyeing, plastics, hairdressing, bakery, dry cleaning and metal industries, to name a few.
Those in the rubber industry are at increasing risk due to

Some common contact allergens

- nickel
- chromium
- thimerosal
- formaldehyde
- p-phenylenediamine
- balsam of Peru
- cinnamic alcohol, cinnamic aldehyde
- p-tertiary-butylphenol formaldehyde resin
- latex rubber, latex additives

- plants – such as poison ivy, poison sumac, chrysanthemum
- topical medications such as neomycin, benzocaine, corticosteroids
- ethylenediamine dihydrochloride
- cosmetic stabilizers, fragrances
- soaps, hair dyes, aftershave lotion
- antimicrobials (in soaps, toothpaste, moisturizing lotions)

additives in rubber products, and healthcare workers often react to the latex in rubber gloves (see below).

Also at risk are people with hobbies that involve sensitizing substances. Allergy-prone gardeners sometimes develop "tulip fingers," or primula or nasturtium dermatitis. Artists may develop allergic contact dermatitis from their paints, and model builders may become allergic to the glues and resins they use.

Cosmetic products are notorious for causing contact dermatitis. A recent report detailed vulval contact dermatitis in some women who used Always sanitary napkins. The symptoms, first wrongly attributed to vaginitis or a yeast infection, were found to occur during or just after the woman's period (in contrast to vaginitis, which is most frequent between periods). In some cases the dermatitis exactly followed the napkin outline. Changing the brand of sanitary napkin abolished the problem. (Although allergies to perfumed products are common, Always napkins are perfume-free, and the vulvar irritation may be due to another component.)

Contact dermatitis is not common in infancy, because of

lack of exposure and immune-system immaturity. Children most commonly develop contact dermatitis to drugs (such as antibiotics), shoes and clothing, perfumed products or poison ivy. One child developed a contact allergy to crayons; another developed latex dermatitis from chewing erasers. In one typical case, a 19-year-old who had never been allergic to anything took a job as a hairdressing assistant. Soon after she started the job, her hands became covered with a rash that refused to clear with any medications or creams. Patch testing showed that she had developed a contact allergy to hair dyes, worsened by irritant soaps and shampoos. She tried wearing rubber gloves to keep her problem under control, but the contact dermatitis persisted and she had to change jobs.

How Contact Dermatitis Begins

People generally become sensitized by direct contact with the substance, and more than one exposure is often required. The allergens that trigger contact dermatitis are typically *haptens*

Nickel is a frequent culprit

One of the few population surveys of contact dermatitis ever conducted, a 1979 San Francisco study, found that about 6 percent of the volunteers were sensitized to nickel. Nickel is commonly used in jewelry, coins, zippers, clasps, buttons and a myriad of other products. Earrings are a common cause of nickel sensitivity. Girls are (or used to be) more likely than boys to have their ears pierced and become nickel-sensitive. In one Swedish study of schoolgirls aged 8 to 15 years, 15 percent of those with pierced ears were nickel-sensitive, compared to 2 percent of boys. However, as fashions change and more teenage boys have their ears, noses, navels and other body parts pierced, nickel allergy is beginning to increase among them. The chance of nickel sensitivity rises with the number of pierced holes. A Finnish study found 35 percent of girls with more than one ear piercing hypersensitive to nickel, compared to 15 percent of those with only one piercing.

(very small molecules), which are too small to stimulate an allergic reaction themselves but do so by "piggybacking" on skin proteins. The immunological mechanism involved is a type IV delayed reaction involving T-cells, although type I IgE reactions can also occur to certain chemicals.

Initial sensitization usually requires a larger amount of chemical exposure but, once sensitized, the person can react to tiny amounts of the allergen, developing symptoms at each contact and usually remaining sensitive for life. A roadworker who works day after day with cement, or a dentist who wears latex gloves for hours every day, is more likely to become sensitized than someone with only occasional contact. Sometimes, as with latex, the product can not only trigger a local skin reaction but – if particles become airborne and are inhaled – provoke a generalized IgE-mediated reaction, even life-threatening anaphylaxis.

Contact dermatitis can affect any part of the body, but most frequently attacks the hands and face or areas where the skin is thin. Eyelid skin, for instance, is thinner than that on the rest of the face, so certain products may affect the eyelids but cause no face rash. Neck and genital areas are also thin and likely to develop dermatitis. Untreated, contact dermatitis can become very itchy, dry and scaly. If the rash becomes infected with bacteria, a more severe condition can develop.

Once someone is sensitized, the rash typically appears 12 to 48 hours after contact with the offending allergen, and lasts a few days to weeks. In the acute stage there is an inflamed, itchy, burning rash, and there may be blisters. Contact dermatitis around the loose skin of the eyes can cause painful swelling. Symptoms usually clear up if the person stops being exposed to the aggravating trigger. In some cases of occupational dermatitis the skin rash does not completely clear even after the person quits the allergy-provoking work, and occasionally the condition becomes chronic.

Making a Diagnosis

To diagnose contact dermatitis, it must be distinguished from other conditions easily confused with it, such as eczema, seborrhea (a greasy, yellowish rash on the scalp and elsewhere) and irritant dermatitis (which is hard to distinguish from allergic dermatitis).

Finding the allergen responsible can be tricky. Your physician will take a detailed history, asking about your job, your kind of work, products you encounter on the job, recent changes in your workplace and any cosmetics you use. You may also be asked about your hobbies.

The site of the rash gives hints about the cause: a bracelet shape on the wrist or a sandal-strap shape on the foot clearly points to a metal allergy or to leather dermatitis. A young man who developed a strange rash around his mouth turned out to be allergic to his fiancée's lipstick. A night watchman who developed eyelid dermatitis was found to be allergic to the brass cleaner used on the building's brass doorknobs; apparently he rubbed his eyes with contaminated hands. In another case, a man with dermatitis on his thighs turned out to be nickel-allergic to the keys in his pocket.

- *Eyelid dermatitis* is commonly traced to mascara, eye shadow or other eye make-up and eye-grooming articles. One woman with nickel sensitivity developed eyelid dermatitis from her metal eyelash curler. Another woman got it from nail polish, after rubbing her eyes with her fingernails – a common form of eye dermatitis.
- *Scalp dermatitis* can arise from hair dyes, permanent-wave solutions, sprays or conditioners. Changing brands can solve the problem.

- *Earlobe dermatitis* often comes from jewelry, perfumes or cosmetics.
- *Face and neck dermatitis* often stems from hair dyes, make-up, perfume, soaps or creams, as well as cosmetic sponges, brushes, grooming aids or mouthwashes.
- *Underarm contact dermatitis* can arise from deodorants, dress shields, dry-cleaning fluids, fabric softeners or simply detergent residue in clothing.
- *Dermatitis in the genital area* may stem from scented or colored toilet paper, or sanitary napkins, douches or condoms – even if these are a partner's products.
- A *skin allergy* on the feet may point to foot powders, shoe leathers, or footwear cleaners.

If, after careful history-taking, the reason for the dermatitis remains elusive, patch tests may provide the answer. The products to be tested are put on the skin of the back in a row, and the spots are covered with protective patches. After 48 hours the patches are lifted; the skin beneath is inspected then and rechecked at 96 hours, as some substances cause delayed reactions. An itchy, red, raised spot at the application site denotes sensitivity to the product tested. A strong allergic reaction may produce an uncomfortable rash under the patch. In some cases, allergy tests are done on a person's entire range of cosmetics, to try to pinpoint the one causing the dermatitis. Patch-test results must be interpreted by a skilled allergy expert, but even a positive result is not necessarily proof of a contact allergen.

Drawbacks to the patch test are that it is time-consuming, requires three office visits and doesn't give foolproof answers. But patch tests are accepted as valid for claims by insurance companies and worker-compensation boards for adverse reactions on the job. Once the allergic trigger has been found, avoiding it is the best solution, if possible.

Managing Contact Dermatitis

Allergic contact rashes are treated in two stages. For the acute blistery stage, compresses are used. The affected area is compressed for five to seven minutes by a cold compress or a washcloth soaked in a solution recommended by a dermatologist, and then wrung out, several times a day. For more extensive dermatitis, bathing may bring relief, but don't soak for too long. Some dermatologists recommend adding Burow's solution (aluminum acetate) to the bathwater. Once the blisters have dried, a corticosteroid cream can reduce the inflammation and clear the rash. For widespread or severe dermatitis, oral steroids may be prescribed.

When the triggering agent has been traced and the rash has cleared, preventing future outbreaks can be difficult. Some allergens are so widespread that they are hard to avoid, and some are integral to the work environment. Whether quitting the job will clear the dermatitis depends on the type of allergen causing it. For instance, people allergic to epoxy resins (as in glues) usually do well when they stop working with the substance; those sensitized to glutaraldehyde, a common disinfectant in dentists' offices, are more likely to have ongoing dermatitis, and an occupationally developed latex allergy can continue to create problems long after the employee leaves the workplace.

Poison Ivy Dermatitis

"Berries three, better flee
Berries white, a poisonous sight."

Although many people think of poison ivy as being harmful to everyone, in fact the reaction to it is allergic. Of those who stumble into a patch of poison ivy on a hike, at the cottage or on a farm, only about 85 percent are affected. The poison ivy plant is a member of the cashew family and grows coast to coast in North America, though in some areas it's called "poison oak." Poison sumac, which also grows across the continent, is closely related and has similar effects. In those already sensitized, a poison ivy rash usually breaks out within 12 to 48 hours of contact, as an inflamed, itchy – often blistered – eruption marking the plant's contact with the body, often with streaks on the legs or arms. The rash appears wherever the poison ivy leaves touched the skin, and wherever ivy-contaminated hands or clothes touched the skin.

The potent allergenic substance in poison ivy, urushiol, is present in the plant's sap and oil, in the stem, roots and leaves. Poison ivy can cause a rash even if the dead leaves are touched in winter, or if the fur of contaminated pets is touched, or a ball or other toy that has rolled into the plants. You can get an outbreak if you don contaminated clothes – even months or a year later. The rash can last days to weeks, and may become very severe if not promptly treated.

Take 19-year-old Joanna, a visiting nanny from Germany. She and the family that employed her went on a picnic and sat in a patch of poison ivy. A day later the entire family – mother, father and all three children – broke out in a poison ivy rash. But Joanna had no rash. Because she was from Europe, where poison ivy doesn't grow, she had never become sensitized to it. But the second time she accidentally encountered it, a year later on a canoe trip, she developed a fearsomely itchy rash within 24 hours. Far from medical aid, she used calamine lotion to soothe the itch. When she sought medical attention a few days later, the physician chided her for having left the rash unattended and prescribed a course of steroid tablets.

The treatment for poison ivy is topical corticosteroid creams, and often oral steroids for severe cases. Antihistamines can help to reduce the itching. Keep the blisters clean

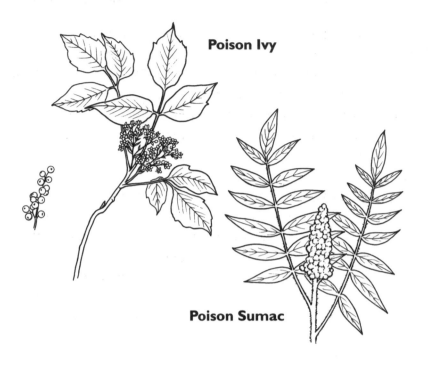

Poison Ivy

Poison Sumac

and apply cold compresses or ice packs. Aluminum acetate (Burow's) solution, applied for five to ten minutes every few hours, can help dry out the blisters. Bathing with oatmeal (Aveeno) can bring relief.

Unfortunately most people don't know they have encountered the noxious plant until they break out in the rash. The best remedy for poison ivy is prevention and avoidance – learning to recognize the plant's three droopy, shiny, lobed leaves in a spreading vine or shrub. If your neighborhood harbors poison ivy, consider posting a color photograph of the plant so that children and visitors can spot it and avoid it.

After touching poison ivy, wash the plant oil from the skin as soon as possible with soap and water, taking care not to spread the oil farther. If the oil is washed off within twenty minutes, only a mild rash (or none) may appear. Even after a few hours, thorough washing with soap (not forgetting to wash under fingernails, rings and watchbands) or rubbing alcohol can lessen the reaction. Alcohol-soaked cleansing pads are effective, and dabbing calamine on affected parts can soothe the itch. Contaminated clothing should be washed in hot water and detergent. If you suspect your pet got into the plant, wash it too!

Tips for Controlling Allergic Contact Dermatitis
- Minimize or avoid contact with sensitizing allergens.
- Always wear gloves when using solvents, thinners, polishes, adhesives, glues or other possible allergens.
- Wear cotton gloves for dry, dusty or dirty work (such as housework, gardening).
- Don't wear rings when doing housework (to avoid rubbing).
- When outdoors in cold or windy weather, wear gloves to protect your hands from drying and chapping.
- Purchase unscented products, including paper products.
- Be wary of products labeled "hypoallergenic." Many hypoallergenic products can cause reactions.
- Use cotton-lined vinyl gloves for activities involving strong liquids.
- Use a washing machine and dishwasher whenever possible.

Hand-care Tips
- Limit washing or wetting hands.
- Wash hands in lukewarm or cool water and plain, mild, unscented soap. Rinse well and dry gently. Then apply lubricant and massage in well.
- Keep hands well moisturized at all times with protective, fragrance-free cream – preferably types recommended by a dermatologist.

- For dermatitis, apply steroid (cortisone) cream to the hands many times a day – after each hand-washing. Apply it thinly. If desired, the cream can be applied to the whole hand, like a hand cream.
- Do not apply any cream, lotion or ointment to the hands other than the ones prescribed, except for plain white petrolatum (Vaseline).
- When the rash is fading, use steroid cream three to four times a day until the skin has completely healed.

If you have a diagnosed contact allergy, you may need specialist advice in sifting through the modern world of products to find which items contain the offending allergen. For example, formaldehyde is common in paper products, balsam of Peru is common in cosmetics and so on. Also watch for cross-sensitivity. For example, if you are allergic to poison ivy you may react to chemically similar substances such as mangoes and various tree lacquers.

Latex: A Burgeoning New Allergy

Latex has recently become a much-publicized cause of contact allergies, with escalating numbers of serious reactions to latex gloves, condoms and even erasers and balloons. Reports of allergic reactions to latex – a product made from the milky secretions of the rubber tree, *Hevea brasiliensis* – date back almost a century, but only in the late 1970s was it suspected of causing severe reactions. Nowadays latex is found almost anywhere, including bicycle handgrips, stoppers, hot water bottles, shoe soles, goggles, rubber bands, sports equipment and bandages. Most likely to cause latex sensitization and allergy are thin, dipped products such as latex rubber gloves, balloons and condoms. Molded latex products are less allergy-provoking: toys, tires, escalator hand-rails, shoes and clothing.

Among the general public the risk of an allergic reaction to latex remains below 1 percent, and serious reactions are rare. But the incidence is climbing in healthcare workers, and currently 25 percent of dental workers and 17 percent of other healthcare professionals report latex reactions of varying severity.

Physicians first became alerted to latex allergy when some children who underwent multiple operations to correct spina bifida (an unfused spine) developed a strong allergic reaction during surgery from contact with latex tubing inside the body. Serious latex allergies can occur if surgical gloves and medical tubing touch sensitive inner tissues. Latex is widely used in medical equipment such as catheters, wound drains, syringes and tubing. The so-called epidemic of latex allergies is partly attributed to the increased demand for surgical gloves to prevent disease transmission, which has resulted in less quality control and less carefully manufactured (more allergenic) products.

Latex allergy is provoked by residual proteins from the rubber tree, or by additives used for vulcanization (strengthening). The most common form is a delayed type IV reaction, not usually severe, which peaks 24 to 48 hours after prolonged contact. This type of allergy causes a local reaction, generally a rash or eczema at the point of contact. If it's due to rubber gloves, the eczema appears on the hands. Women may develop vaginal irritation and itching if their partners wear latex condoms.

The less usual form of latex allergy is a type I, IgE-antibody reaction from direct contact or from inhaling airborne particles. The powder used inside surgical gloves spreads the latex protein into the air, where it can cause severe reactions, even anaphylaxis. In operating rooms and dental offices, where pre-powdered gloves are many times donned and removed, someone with a latex allergy may breathe in latex proteins and react suddenly and severely. If you are allergic to latex, warn your healthcare providers of your vulnerability.

Although it has long been known that latex can cause contact rashes, allergic shock and death from this product were almost unknown before reports trickled in during the late 1980s. At a conference in 1988, researchers reported the case of a Toronto operating-room nurse who collapsed and nearly died from an anaphylactic reaction to latex rubber. Physicians and nurses with this allergy may have to give up activities that require them to wear latex gloves, or stop working in latex-laden environments.

Use of non-powdered, "low-protein" gloves may be the solution. In one case, a switch by all co-workers to powder-free latex gloves allowed an allergic employee to keep her job. But finding alternatives for latex is a problem, as other materials are less flexible, split more easily and cost more. Moreover, gloves made of alternative products such as vinyl are more permeable to blood and water, and may be more apt to allow infectious agents through – though this is less likely with more expensive substitutes such as neoprene. Manufacturers are now trying to make latex products lower in rubber-tree proteins.

Some people with latex allergy develop an itchy mouth when they eat bananas, avocados, kiwi fruit or chestnuts, which contain proteins resembling those of the rubber tree. The sap of the houseplant *Ficus benjamina* (weeping fig) can trigger allergic reactions in latex-sensitive people.

Unusual cases of latex allergy include a woman married to a physician, who suffered severe wheezing in response to traces of latex on her husband's clothing; he had to change his clothes and wash thoroughly as soon as he came home from the hospital. Another woman developed a serious latex reaction to the grip on her squash racket. Fast-food workers often wear rubber gloves while preparing meals, and latex-sensitive customers have collapsed after eating latex-contaminated sandwiches and chicken dinners.

Contact Dermatitis and the Consumer

The law in Canada does not require that non-foods such as cosmetics and textiles be labeled with their contents, so you can't always know if you are being exposed to a specific allergen. In the U.S., labeling on many non-food items is very detailed, and includes such ingredients as colors, fragrances, thickeners and others. However, even when products are labeled or ingredients are listed, you may be lost in what one writer called a "synonymic jungle." Many chemicals have so many synonyms that it's hard to recognize all their names. If possible, get involved in pushing for better labeling laws, with full disclosure of all product ingredients. Most improvements in consumer information come about because consumers themselves insist on knowing what they are putting in, on and around their bodies.

THIRTEEN

Eye Allergies

Eye (ocular) allergies, causing red, itchy, runny eyes, affect about 15 per cent of the North American population from time to time. They range from the seasonal "allergic conjunctivitis" that often accompanies hay fever or a mold allergy to more severe forms such as one that parallels atopic dermatitis (eczema) – one of the very few eye allergies that may scar and damage the eye's clear outer covering, or *cornea*.

Eye allergies chiefly involve the *conjunctiva* – a thin membrane over the white parts of the eye, extending inside the eyelids, that's richly supplied with blood vessels and mast cells. As with other allergies, it's the mediators released from the mast cells that produce the allergic symptoms. Normally both eyes become red, watery and itchy, but occasionally only one eye is affected – perhaps because that eye has been rubbed with a finger contaminated with some allergy-provoking material. "One eye allergy we often see," notes a Californian ophthalmologist (eye doctor), "comes from rubbing the eye with nail polish, or another freshly applied, allergenic nail product."

Anatomy of the Eye

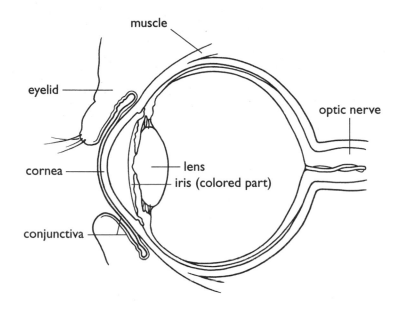

Like other allergies, IgE-mediated ocular allergies are due to immune-system activity: IgE antibodies, formed in response to an allergen touching the eye, provoke the cascade of allergic events. Mast cells in the eye's conjunctiva degranulate and release potent mediators such as the histamine and others already described, producing the itching, inflammation, teariness and swelling.

Eye Allergies Rarely Occur Alone

Eye allergies usually accompany another allergic condition, even though the affected person may not realize that the two are linked. However, it can take more of a provocative allergen to cause eye symptoms than nasal discomfort, since – although the eye is an open surface – blinking and tears wash away some of the offending substances.

Generally more irritating and uncomfortable than serious,

eye allergies are very often linked to seasonal or year-round rhinitis, which is why allergists like to call the condition "rhinoconjunctivitis" – denoting both eye and nose symptoms. The same pollens that cause hay fever, or the cat dander responsible for a pet allergy, can also cause allergic eye discomfort. But a few ocular allergies occur without nasal symptoms, and some can be severe and require the prompt attention of an eye specialist.

Recognizing an Eye Allergy

Many people realize they have an eye allergy when the redness, itching and tearing start up as soon as the hay fever season hits, or when discomfort begins right after an animal enters the room. Eye allergies can be diagnosed through taking the medical history, asking about the nature of the eye symptoms, when they occur, any associated nasal discomfort, the work situation, family background and any other allergies the person may have, such as atopic dermatitis or asthma.

Eyes that look "milky," red and inflamed strongly suggest an allergy, as do upper eyelids that are swollen and droopy. The eye specialist may detect changes in the conjunctiva, perhaps profuse mast cells, and definite signs of inflammation in the conjunctiva. (A brilliantly red eye with a discharge of pus is more typical of a bacterial eye infection than an allergy.)

The tears may contain demonstrably high levels of allergic mediators, such as histamine. Examination of a smear of conjunctival secretions – gently taken from the eye's surface – will often reveal an excess of eosinophils (white cells) if the problem is an allergy. Non-allergic forms of conjunctivitis, such as those due to an irritant or infection, don't raise the eosinophil count.

> ## The hallmarks of eye allergy
> * eye redness, itching and burning
> * watering, "weepiness"
> * swollen eyelids – sometimes an eye swollen shut
> * accompanying rhinitis (nasal stuffiness) and sneezing
> * photophobia (sensitivity to light)
> * "allergic shiners" – bluish smudges around or under both eyes
>   (not to be confused with redness under and around one eye or on
>   the lid, edged by a purple line, due to orbital cellulitis – a medical
>   emergency in children that requires immediate medical attention)

The Five Main Forms of Eye Allergy

* *Allergic rhinoconjunctivitis*, which can be year-round or seasonal (also known as "hay fever conjunctivitis"), accompanying the nasal discomfort of allergic rhinitis, with eye-itching, redness and clear, runny tearing. The pollens that cause seasonal conjunctivitis vary around the world, but the symptoms are the same, and are usually relieved by antihistamines. Year-round allergic conjunctivitis – due to allergy triggers such as molds, dust mites or animal dander – resembles the seasonal form, but is usually milder.

* *Giant papillary conjunctivitis* – an allergy combined with local eye irritation – often a response to local injury, perhaps linked to a foreign body on the eye's surface, or to protein buildup on contact lenses. It is heralded not only by redness and itching but also by a thick mucus discharge. Examination reveals large *papillae* (bumps) on the conjunctiva of the upper eyelid.

* *Atopic keratoconjunctivitis (AKC)* – among the most serious of ocular allergies. (*Kerato* means "pertaining to the cornea.") It usually begins during adolescence, and may accompany eczema lingering on from childhood. This

allergy is characterized by intense itching, a heavy eye discharge, vision blurring and skin changes in the eyelids. There may be severe conjunctival inflammation, possibly involving the cornea and causing vision problems.

- *Vernal keratoconjunctivitis* – a rare but incapacitating seasonal allergy in both eyes, seen mainly in young people. This typically starts in spring ("vernal" means "spring") and may last through summer. Often it appears at puberty and is gone by adulthood. The eyes are red, itchy and light-sensitive, with a stringy discharge, droopy lids and enlarged papillae inside the upper eyelids. A family or personal history of allergies is often present. An eye exam reveals severe inflammation, numerous mast cells and telltale eosinophils. Treatment may require corticosteroids.

- *Contact eye allergies*, which stem from a wide array of products (including contact-lens solutions and eye medications), causing redness, intense itching, tearing and swelling. They may accompany dermatitis due to skin contact with an allergy-triggering agent such as latex, poison ivy or a cosmetic ingredient. Mascara, eyebrow pencil and eye creams are notoriously troublesome. Rubbing the eyes after handling soaps, nail polish, detergents or other allergy-causing chemicals often triggers an acute contact eye allergy.

Managing Eye Allergies

Therapy resembles that for other allergic problems: avoid the provocative allergens if possible, and use antihistamines and other medications to relieve the discomfort. Cold compresses put on the eye several times a day often help. Many people with an eye allergy manage the condition quite well on their own, using one or more recommended over-the-counter products, usually as eyedrops.

Combination eyedrops, containing an antihistamine and a vasoconstrictor, lessen the itch, take away the redness and whiten the eyes (by constricting blood vessels). For mild cases, antihistamine-vasoconstrictor drops are often enough – for example, antazoline or levocabastine combined with a topical vasoconstrictor such as naphazoline. Most are used two to four times a day, and side-effects are minimal unless use is very prolonged.

Antihistamine tablets may also help to relieve the eye discomfort.

Cromolyn and lodoxamide eyedrops (mast-cell stabilizers, to stop the release of mediators) may be added, and NSAIDs (non-steroidal anti-inflammatory drugs) such as ketorolac (Acular) and rimexolone can also be helpful. Cromolyn compounds (e.g., Opticrom, Cromolon) are usually tried before NSAIDs or corticosteroids. Unlike corticosteroids, cromolyn and NSAIDs have minimal side-effects; as an extra plus, cromolyn reduces nasal congestion.

Topical corticosteroids, usually as drops, are considered backup medications, to be used only if other medications don't work. They should be taken under close medical supervision as their side-effects could damage the eye.

Systemic corticosteroids, although rarely necessary, are occasionally prescribed for severe cases – for example, poison ivy that attacks the eyes.

Immunotherapy – injection of specific allergen extracts – can be effective for eye symptoms related to hay fever.

As a word of caution, one eye doctor warns that "combined anti-inflammatory (steroid) plus antibiotic drops should *never* be automatically taken or prescribed without medical supervision as corticosteroids wrongly used can injure the eyes."

Medical advice should be obtained promptly if there is a lot of pain, extreme eye redness or a heavy discharge, or if the problem doesn't respond to over-the-counter medication. Quite often an infection occurs alongside the allergy, requiring appropriate antibiotics.

Especially Useful Anti-allergy Eye Medications

- *levocabastine* (Livostin) – a potent local antihistamine
- *vasoconstrictors* – many are available in non-prescription

Medications for Eye Allergies

Generic name	Some brand names	Formulation	Action
Antazoline	Albalon-A, Vasocon-A	drops	antihistamine-vasoconstrictor (also contains naphazoline)
Astemizole	Hismanal	tablets	antihistamine
Cromolyn/ cromoglycate	Opticrom, Rynacrom, Vistacrom†	drops, ointment	mast-cell stabilizer
Dexamethasone	Decadron, Ocudex†	drops, tablets	corticosteroid anti-inflammatory
Fluorometholone	FML, FML-Forte	drops	corticosteroid
Ketorolac	Acular, Toradol	drops	nonsteroidal anti-inflammatory
Levocabastine	Livostin	drops	antihistamine
Lodoxamide	Alomide	drops	mast-cell stabilizer
Naphazoline	Naphcon, Vasocon	drops	vasoconstrictor
Prednisolone	Delta-Cortef, Ocu-Pred	drops	corticosteroid anti-inflammatory
Prednisone	Deltasone, Meticorten	tablets	corticosteroid
Rimexolone	Vexol*	drops	corticosteroid
Terfenadine	Seldane	tablets	antihistamine
Tetrahydrozoline	Visine	drops	vasoconstrictor
Xylometazoline-antazoline	Ophtrivin-A	eyedrops†, nose spray*	vasoconstrictor-antihistamine

*Available in U.S. only.
†Available in Canada only.

Eyedrops with corticosteroids must be used sparingly as they can cause glaucoma and cataracts. Use only with a physician's supervision.

forms, for instance naphazoline (in Vasocon-A and Naphcon)

- *ketorolac* (Acular), a nonsteroidal anti-inflammatory and potent itch-reliever
- *lodoxamide* (Alomide), a mast-cell stabilizer – very effective in controlling vernal and giant papillary eye allergies

Use Eyedrops in Moderation – Especially Steroids

Conjunctivitis medicamentosa is a term used to describe problems caused by excess use of eye medications, especially vasoconstrictor drops – "not usually ones prescribed by an eye doctor," notes one renowned ophthalmologist. "It can also arise from preservatives in artificial tears, glaucoma drops, antibiotic preparations and contact-lens solutions." Eye preparations containing neomycin, atropine and its derivatives, and thimerosal are also frequent allergy-provokers. Typically, once the eyedrops are used, symptoms improve, but as the medication is continued the eyes again become red and itchy. More drops (or perhaps different eye preparations) are tried, starting a vicious cycle of inflammation. The eyes stay red and weepy, the eyelids swollen. It's hard to tell whether the problem stems from the original complaint or from the medication. The best idea is to stop taking the eyedrops; many cases clear up once all eye medication is given up. If the conjunctivitis is due to necessary drugs such as neomycin, atropine or sulfacetamide, the best strategy is to substitute other, non-irritating medications.

"Topical corticosteroids should be used with the greatest caution," adds one eye specialist, "always under medical supervision, and usually just for a brief course, as cortisone in the eyes increases the risk of cataracts, glaucoma and corneal infections. They should be used for the shortest possible time, in low doses." These anti-inflammatories can quickly relieve an eye allergy, but since the problem is often ongoing or recurrent they are usually recommended only in severe cases. If they are needed for longer than a week or so, internal eye pressure should be measured before starting corticosteroid therapy, and once a month thereafter.

"Under no circumstances," stresses the specialist, "should people use corticosteroid eyedrops without medical monitoring." To minimize the dose, the corticosteroid can be added to other preparations, rather than replacing them. Before someone is given topical corticosteroids, herpes simplex conjunctivitis should be ruled out, because steroids aggravate and spread herpes infections.

FOURTEEN

While the arsenal of medications now available to remedy our ailments brings untold benefits, it also brings some risks. Undesirable reactions can occur with both prescribed and over-the-counter products. People often diagnose themselves as allergic to this or that medication, when in fact the problem is usually not an allergy but a predictable, non-immunological side-effect – for instance, headache, bloating, nausea or diarrhea. Only a small proportion – about 6 to 12 percent – of all adverse reactions to drugs are allergic, but they tend to be among the more severe reactions. A few drugs cause both non-allergic and allergic reactions. To help you distinguish one from the other, we will first look at non-allergic reactions.

Non-allergic Adverse Drug Reactions

Most adverse reactions are predictable side-effects, or stem from intolerance or overdose (toxicity). Hardly any medications are completely devoid of side-effects, and all drugs, even vitamins and other health supplements, should be kept well out of the reach of children, preferably in locked cabinets.

Predictable Adverse Reactions

- *Toxicity* results from taking amounts that exceed the recommended dose for your age, sex and weight.

- *Known side-effects* are due to biological changes that accompany the medication's desired therapeutic effects. These can be unpleasant, occasionally detrimental, and if they are severe they should be reported to a physician. Side-effects are listed on the drug package or bottle, and for prescription medications your doctor may warn you about side-effects that could be especially troublesome or pose a risk. Pharmacists are also knowledgeable sources of information.

- *Secondary effects* are those not directly linked to the drug's primary action. For example, use of certain antibiotics may alter the natural balance of bacteria in the bowel, producing diarrhea. Regular use of corticosteroid inhalers (e.g., for asthma or hay fever) can lead to a yeast overgrowth in the mouth.

- *Drug/drug and drug/food interactions* can also alter the action and efficacy of medications – one reason why your physician may ask about all the drugs you are taking. Certain medications that are safe when taken alone can produce severe adverse reactions when taken at the same time as another drug or a certain food. MAO inhibitors react adversely with certain cheeses; the antihistamine terfenadine can cause heart disturbances in combination with certain antifungals; cimetidine (a stomach ulcer drug) can increase the effect of some anticonvulsants (e.g., phenytoin); some cold remedies can alter the efficacy of anti-diabetes pills – the list is endless. *The key to avoiding these reactions is to read labels carefully!*

Unpredictable Adverse Reactions

Although these account for less than one-fifth of all adverse responses, they are among the most hazardous, as they're unexpected and can be severe. They arise from biochemical differences that make some people unable to handle certain medications even in small doses.

- *Drug intolerances* cause an exaggeratedly severe side-effect or other reaction that may resemble the effects of an overdose of the drug – for example, tinnitus, or ringing in the ears, from an average ASA (aspirin) dose, or vomiting after taking erythromycin, which usually causes only mild diarrhea.

- *Drug idiosyncrasies* can be due to an inherited biochemical change that produces an abnormal reaction. Knowing that other family members have responded in a similar manner can be a forewarning. For instance, some people of Mediterranean or African descent lack the enzyme glucose-6-phosphate dehydrogenase in their red blood cells, making them unable to metabolize certain sulfa and ASA-containing drugs, so that even small amounts can produce severe blood problems. (The enzyme lack can be detected by a simple blood test so these people can avoid the troublesome drugs.) Similarly a drug idiosyncrasy may lead to hepatitis from common anticonvulsants, or to Stevens-Johnson syndrome (a severe skin reaction) in response to sulfonamides.

Drug Allergies

Like other allergies, drug allergies are immunological reactions, usually involving IgE antibodies and the release of mediators from T-cells. They produce a set of specific and recognizable symptoms ranging from hives, swelling and

> ## "Drug allergies" that aren't
>
> About 10 to 15 percent of people think they are allergic to certain drugs such as penicillin, but skin tests show that three-quarters of those who believe themselves allergic to penicillin are not, in fact, allergic to it. People who wrongly believe they are allergic to a drug may not be offered (or may refuse to take) the best remedy for an ailment. For example, people who imagine they are allergic to local anesthetics used by dentists must either endure tooth pain when they have drilling, or accept stronger, possibly hazardous painkillers. Check out supposed allergies with an allergist before limiting your treatment options.

itching to life-threatening anaphylaxis – unlike the various symptoms of non-allergic drug reactions. Allergic drug reactions span a wider range of immunological responses than many other allergies, and in addition to IgE reactions they include serum sickness, drug fever, autoimmune reactions and "pseudoallergies" – due to direct mediator release from mast cells.

Allergy-provoking Drugs: It's a Long List

Allergic drug reactions are among the most common causes of life-endangering allergic shock; they are less frequent in the elderly than in younger adults. Penicillin is among the most frequent causes of anaphylaxis seen in hospital emergency departments. Other antibiotics known to cause allergies, sometimes severe, include the cephalosporins, sulfa drugs, chloramphenicol, clindamycin, aminoglycosides and some antifungals. In one large collaborative U.S study, the most common and serious drug allergies were to penicillin and its relatives, followed by sulfonamides and cephalosporins. A few people have multiple antibiotic allergies.

The list of other medications that can cause allergic (or "allergy-like") reactions includes: ASA and other nonsteroidal anti-inflammatories (NSAIDs), opiates such as codeine and morphine, anesthetics, streptokinase (a clot-dissolving drug), hormones such as pig-derived insulin, various anticonvulsants, muscle relaxants, heparin (a blood thinner), gamma globulin and radiocontrast dyes (used in X-ray imaging).

Cross-reactivity can occur with drugs: people allergic to one medication may be allergic to others with a similar chemical structure. For example, if you're allergic to one anticonvulsant you may also react to some others. If you're allergic to one form of penicillin you may react not only to other forms of penicillin but also to cephalosporins, which share molecular similarities with penicillin. If you're allergic to sulfonamides you may also react to other sulfa-based medications such as sulfonylureas (used to control blood sugar).

Drug-sensitization Takes Time

As with other allergies, most people do not have an allergic reaction the first time they take a certain medication, because it takes a few days to several weeks after first exposure to become "sensitized." Sometimes people have been sensitized to a drug they have never knowingly taken – for example, to penicillin in cow's milk, beef or veal – and are amazed at the swift and dramatic symptoms that hit them "out of the blue."

Once they are sensitized, those who are allergic can react to even traces of the drug, sometimes with a sudden, severe and unexpected response – perhaps even anaphylactic shock.

The first allergic episode often appears when someone has been on a certain drug for a week to ten days – and may even happen a little while after the drug is stopped. Symptoms can appear within minutes of taking the medication again, or a few hours or days later. A "late phase" reaction, as bad as the first or worse, can follow some hours later.

Most drug molecules are too small to activate the immune system directly, but their particles can combine with body proteins to create a *hapten-carrier* combination, or "combination immunogen." For example, one woman developed hives, skin itching and swelling two weeks after going off the antibiotic Ceclor. The reaction was not identified as a drug allergy. The second time she took Ceclor the hives and other symptoms developed at the end of the ten-day drug course, and again were not recognized as an allergic response. The third time she took the drug, a year later, she broke out in hives within 24 hours. The physician at the hospital emergency department spotted the problem as an allergy, and warned her to stay off Ceclor and related drugs in future.

Medications are most likely to induce allergies if they are taken as several short courses in swift succession – for example, when an infection recurs. Injected drugs tend to be more allergy-provoking than those taken by mouth. Medications put on the skin can also provoke allergic reactions, with a rash and swelling. Anyone who has had a severe drug reaction should take preventive precautions, as the same drug may produce similar or even more severe symptoms next time around. People with other allergies – for instance, a food allergy, eczema or inhalant allergies such as mold allergies or hay fever, are *not* more susceptible to a drug allergy. However, those with the "allergic triad" – asthma, sinusitis and nose polyps – are at greater risk of allergy to ASA and other NSAIDs. People allergic to one drug are often at elevated risk of other, even unrelated drug allergies.

The risk of severe drug reactions and anaphylaxis increases in people taking beta-blocker medications, partly because beta blockers block the effects of epinephrine, making allergic anaphylaxis very hard to treat.

Allergic and Allergy-like Reactions Vary
Drug allergies include several types of immunological reaction,

as well as "pseudoallergic" reactions. Allergic drug responses may be immediate, type I, IgE-mediated reactions, which usually start within minutes to an hour of taking the drug (see Chapter Two); non-IgE immune-system reactions may take longer to surface. The same drug can cause a variety of allergic and pseudoallergic reactions. Penicillin, for instance, can cause IgE-mediated, rapid-onset anaphylaxis as well as different immune-complex reactions, often accompanied by fever – known as a "serum sickness–like" response (see below).

Type II or "cytotoxic" drug reactions are toxic (poisonous) to the body's own cells, and occur if drugs attach to and attack certain cells. This can happen with penicillin, quinidine and some other drugs, producing hemolytic anemia, which destroys the body's red blood cells.

Type III or immune-complex drug allergies cause serum sickness, with fever and flu-like malaise.

Delayed or type IV drug reactions surface 10 to 20 days after exposure, and involve activated T-lymphocytes. They often cause contact dermatitis. They occur from many products, such as those containing the antibiotics neomycin and bacitracin, or sunscreens containing para-aminobenzoic acid (PABA). Occasionally, delayed drug reactions affect the lungs, as can happen with the anticonvulsants phenytoin and nitrofurantoin. The mechanisms underlying these reactions are still poorly understood.

Symptoms of Drug Allergy

The symptoms are like those of other allergies, with a rash, hives (sometimes huge) and red skin blotches as frequent warning signs. There may also be skin flushing, swelling, nausea, nasal congestion, a swollen larynx and, in serious cases, difficulty breathing. A severe but rare non-allergic skin condition known as "Stevens-Johnson syndrome" – with peeling, blistering, ulcerating dermatitis – can accompany a drug allergy, confusing the picture. Unlike most allergies, allergic drug reactions can include fever as well. The fever may also occur alone – with no other allergic symptoms, no rash or hives – and so can be hard to distinguish from a feverish illness for which the drug has been prescribed.

Pseudoallergic Drug Reactions

Some non-allergic drug reactions closely mimic IgE-triggered allergies, and are as serious, but have different mechanisms. Opiate drugs (such as codeine) can cause symptoms identical to anaphylaxis – with swelling of the tongue and throat, flushing, hives, troubled breathing and allergic shock. But in this case the histamine release occurs through *direct*, non-IgE stimulation of mast cells, rather than through an antibody mechanism. Since such reactions resemble allergic symptoms, they are called *pseudoallergic reactions*.

Anaphylactoid Drug Reactions Mimic Anaphylaxis

These reactions are immunological events mediated by the drug's direct action on mast cells, triggering the release of histamine – without the intervention of IgE antibodies. Even though these reactions are not IgE-linked, they can lead to anaphylaxis with equal rapidity and be just as life-threatening. In this case they are called "anaphylactoid responses." Anaphylactoid responses can arise from a variety of medications such as codeine, morphine, vancomycin (an antibiotic) and niacin (vitamin B_3). They may be suspected when someone never before exposed to a drug collapses suddenly. Although anaphylactoid reactions have a different mechanism, they are treated exactly like anaphylaxis – with epinephrine injection and hospital surveillance.

Radiocontrast materials used in certain X-ray examinations

are well-known causes of anaphylactoid reactions. Injected into the bloodstream, the dyes are used to reveal defects in certain organs – such as the heart and coronary arteries – before a bypass operation or other surgery. About 2 percent of people who receive radiocontrast dyes are at risk of an anaphylactoid reaction, which can occur without any warning and can be severe. Unfortunately, skin tests do not reliably predict who's sensitive to these materials. People with allergic tendencies or with asthma are at above-average risk. The risk of a repeat anaphylactoid reaction to radiocontrast dyes can be reduced if the person is given steroids (prednisone) and antihistamines some hours before the X-ray examination, or if alternative contrast media are used. Newer radiocontrast agents are being developed that are less likely to cause such reactions.

Serum Sickness: A Drug Allergy with Fever
"Serum sickness," a type III (immune-complex) allergy, is a reaction in which the drug-antibody complex causes fever, inflammation, malaise, swollen lymph nodes, puffy hands and feet, swelling of the face, eyelids and lips, and pervasive joint aches. It usually surfaces 7 to 21 days after someone starts a particular drug – sometimes sooner. Unlike most allergic reactions, it can develop the first time a medication is taken, without previous sensitization. About 60 percent of such reactions are caused by penicillin, but other drugs can also produce serum sickness – other antibiotics (e.g., sulfonamides, cephalosporins), some sedatives (e.g., barbiturates), phenytoin (an anticonvulsant), isoniazid (a tuberculosis drug), the heart drug digitalis, some diuretics and the tranquilizer chlorpromazine.

For example, a 57-year-old man was admitted to hospital in 1983 for a mysterious illness. During the month before admission he had developed fever, rhinitis and a cough that became increasingly severe, along with chills, muscle aches, weakness and, later, a rash all over his body, and burning hands and tongue. The hospital physicians thought at first that he had an infection, but when the symptoms began to improve as soon as they took the man off his arthritis medication, they suspected a drug reaction. As it turned out, the man had been taking a new NSAID. His symptoms had begun about a month after he'd started on the medication, and they abated as soon as he stopped taking it. His physician diagnosed serum sickness brought on by ketorolac.

Serum sickness is self-limiting and usually lasts only a few days, but may take several weeks to vanish, even once the drug is stopped. Therapy is with antihistamines to relieve the itching, and sometimes corticosteroids (prednisone). This is not the same reaction as *drug fever*, a non-allergic, drug-induced feverish condition with a rash or hives, occasionally due to antibiotics or other drugs.

Diagnosing Drug Allergies Isn't Always Easy

Although some drugs are more apt to cause allergic reactions than others, physicians stress that *any drug* can produce an allergic response. "To complicate matters," says one allergist, "certain diseases cause symptoms similar to an allergy – for example, a rash from a virus infection may resemble that due to an antibiotic allergy – making it hard to come up with the right diagnosis." If you or someone you know seems to be having a drug reaction – even a rash, tingling mouth or slightly swollen tongue – stop taking the medication and get medical attention. If there's any difficulty swallowing, labored breathing or faintness, get to the nearest hospital emergency department at once.

In general, a drug allergy is suspected when there's no other adequate explanation for the reaction, if it differs from known side-effects, if the timing is appropriate and if symptoms strongly suggest an allergy. Referral to an allergist will likely be advised. In diagnosing drug reactions, physicians take a complete history, noting all medications being taken – both prescription and over-the-counter products – the doses, the time lag between starting medications and the onset of symptoms and whether such symptoms have ever before been experienced.

If symptoms appear in someone who has had similar symptoms in the past, and the drug is known to induce allergic reactions, the diagnosis may pose little challenge. However, confirming a drug allergy can be tricky. Drug allergy has been called "the great imitator" because its symptoms are so diverse and so often resemble the disease for which the medication is being taken. And if someone is on many different medications, it can be confusing to try to ferret out the specific drug causing the reaction.

Skin prick tests may be used to detect an IgE-antibody drug allergy, but are useful mainly for penicillin and its derivatives – these are the only drugs for which skin tests have a good record in predicting sensitivity. If a skin prick test is positive for penicillin – that is, if a "weal and flare" develop where the drug was put on the skin – there is a 70 percent chance of a serious reaction should penicillin ever again be taken. A negative penicillin skin test means that in all likelihood the person is not allergic to the drug and can safely take it.

In the absence of reliable skin tests, a drug challenge or "provocation" test may be tried for some medications, especially if the medication is essential. In challenge tests, a very weak solution of the drug is inserted just under the skin. If there's no observed reaction to increasing doses, the drug may be tried by the usual route (perhaps by mouth), again beginning with a minute dose and increasing it gradually to the normal amount. Challenge tests are done just before treatment with the medication, not weeks or months ahead, and must be done in hospital with full emergency equipment close by. They can cause a severe reaction, and should not be done unless the drug in question is the only option for treating an illness, and its benefits outweigh the risks of testing.

Treatment of Drug Allergies

Treatment of a suspected drug allergy is similar to that for other allergies: stop taking the medication, and if anaphylaxis does occur, inject epinephrine. Antihistamines and corticosteroids may be used as well. In very severe cases, the offending drug may be quickly flushed out of the body with intravenous fluids. Alternatives to the allergenic medication may then be suggested.

Desensitizing Injections

When penicillin or some other medication is the only choice for a sick person who is allergic to the drug, once skin tests have verified an allergy, caregivers may recommend desensitizing through immunotherapy. Desensitizing a drug-allergic

---

Most at risk of drug allergies are

- those who have had an allergic drug reaction in the past – they are four to six times as likely to have another reaction as someone who has never before had a reaction to that particular drug
- people who are taking many medications
- people with certain diseases such as lupus erythematosus, cystic fibrosis and Epstein-Barr (mononucleosis) infections
- people with asthma – they have a higher risk of severe drug reactions, especially to ASA, particularly if they also have nasal polyps and sinusitis
- people taking beta blockers

Be cautious with nonprescription drugs too

Over-the-counter drugs should be treated as seriously as prescribed medications; read labels carefully. When discussing health problems with your physician, be sure to report all the medications you're taking – including laxatives, cold remedies, tonics, herbal preparations, suppositories, douches, birth control products and ointments.

---

person means inducing tolerance to the drug (like immunotherapy for insect venoms). Although the tolerance does not always last, the person may tolerate the medication for the period needed to cure the disorder.

Drug immunotherapy is generally done as a speeded-up procedure, taking hours rather than years. The "rush" procedure starts with one ten-thousandth (or less) of the usual dose, and increasingly higher doses are given every 15 minutes over several hours, until a full dose is reached and tolerated. Drug desensitization is usually done in hospital, often in an intensive care unit, in case of an anaphylactic crisis.

Penicillin Allergics

Penicillin is the foremost cause of serious drug-induced allergies – not surprisingly, as penicillin and other antibiotics are among the world's most frequently prescribed medications. Discovered in 1928, penicillin was our first antibiotic (antibiotics are drugs that destroy bacteria). It was originally produced from the mold *Penicillium*, commonly found on moldy bread or in damp basements, but now there are many synthetic forms. (Oddly enough, people allergic to penicillium molds are not necessarily allergic to penicillin.)

An estimated 2 percent of the North American population has some degree of penicillin allergy, including skin reactions, serum sickness and anaphylaxis. Anaphylactic reactions, sometimes fatal, occur in 1 to 5 out of every 10,000 courses prescribed, usually within an hour or two of taking the drug. Severe reactions are more likely if the drug is given by intramuscular or intravenous injection than if it is taken by mouth.

Today's emergency-room personnel are familiar with penicillin reactions. But penicillin only came into widespread use during World War II, and one physician, now retired, recalls his first experience with it, during his residency training at a University of Toronto hospital in 1950. Hospital staff had little experience with drug reactions, and the first report of penicillin death had only just appeared in the medical literature. A woman was rushed into emergency, collapsing with anaphylaxis. As the physician remembers, "It was a very dangerous-looking reaction. What sticks in my mind was her appearance. She was all blown up. Her face was swollen, her tongue was all swollen. Her body was all puffed up. She couldn't breathe. Nowadays we would give her a shot of epinephrine, but then we didn't really know what to do about it. The woman died, as I remember."

These days anyone known to be or suspected of being penicillin-allergic is told not to take any penicillin compounds – and that includes ampicillin, amoxicillin, methicillin, dicloxacillin and pivampicillin, to name a few.

Margaret was 15 years old when she developed an ear infection. Ampicillin was prescribed. After one week on the antibiotic, she broke out in hives, which cleared once she stopped the medication. Many years later, she was once more prescribed ampicillin, for a bacterial throat infection. This time the reaction was immediate. Within 20 minutes of taking her first tablet, she developed hives all over her body, a swollen face and a constricted throat that hampered breathing. She was taken to hospital, where she was at once treated with epinephrine. Doctors identified the root of the anaphylaxis and switched her to another antibiotic.

Although penicillin allergies can last for decades, in some cases the sensitivity fades in five to ten years. Skin testing can determine whether the allergy still persists. As already mentioned, people allergic to penicillin may cross-react with the cephalosporins, so they should not take cephalosporin antibiotics either. There are now many other antibiotics that can be safely used instead, such as

- clindamycin
- vancomycin
- erythromycin
- tetracycline
- clarithromycin

If you're allergic to penicillin, you should wear some form of medical-alert identification, or carry a wallet card clearly stating your allergy, so that you are never given any of this drug family when you are unable to speak for yourself.

But avoidance isn't always that easy; penicillin can show up in unexpected places. Although strict regulations prevent its presence in foods sold in North America, occasional contamination can occur. In one case in the U.S., in 1993, a 74-year-old man's long years of unexplained hives were finally traced to penicillin contamination of the meat he had been purchasing locally. In another case, a 21-year-old woman vacationing in the Canary Islands developed a mysterious itchy rash after a chicken dinner. Overnight, her lips and face began to swell and she began having trouble swallowing – symptoms similar to those of a penicillin reaction she had suffered years before. As the doctor who treated her explained, "In the Canaries, poultry farmers commonly wash their chicken carcasses in penicillin."

Sulfa Allergies

Sulfa drugs are a common class of medications including, for instance, the sulfonamides, such as trimethoprim-sulfamethoxazole (Bactrim), which are widely used antibacterials. About 3 to 6 percent of hospital patients treated with sulfa drugs react adversely to them, with fever, a rash, swollen face, lips and eyelids, and occasionally Stevens-Johnson syndrome. Delayed reaction to sulfa drugs can be serious, and may damage the kidneys, brain or liver. People who react to sulfonamides may also react to other sulfa-based compounds.

ASA and Other NSAID Allergies

Adverse reactions to ASA (also called "aspirin" in the U.S.) and other nonsteroidal anti-inflammatory drugs (NSAIDs) include hives, swelling of the tongue and throat, rhinoconjunctivitis (nasal and eye discomfort), wheezing, breathing difficulties and occasionally anaphylaxis. Some reactions are classic allergic responses, but others are due to drug intolerance or idiosyncrasy. ASA is widely used as a painkiller, fever-reducer and anti-inflammatory agent, and more recently as an anti-clotting ("anti-platelet-aggregation") agent for preventing stroke and heart attack. Immunological reactions to ASA have been recorded for over a century; together with other NSAIDs, ASA accounts for a substantial number of adverse drug reactions.

The hallmarks of an ASA allergy are hives (sometimes giant), swelling, a persistent face flush, eye and nose watering and itching, and perhaps also a mucus discharge, cough, chest tightness and breathing problems. People are designated "ASA sensitive" after they have experienced a skin or respiratory (lung) reaction to ASA. Those with a severe, systemic reaction will likely have similar symptoms whenever they take the drug, but in those with a milder response the allergic reaction may be sporadic and unpredictable. Quite often, taking ASA or other anti-inflammatories aggravates an underlying respiratory condition, or induces "flare-ups," and it often worsens asthma.

An ASA allergy can start at any age, perhaps when someone resumes the medication after a break from taking it. The typical ASA-allergic person is an adult who takes the drug to relieve a cold or bronchitis, then stops, and on taking it again suffers a sudden reaction. The medication may not be suspected as the cause. Medical examination may reveal pale, congested nasal membranes, polyps in the nose, elevated histamine levels and a collection of eosinophils (white cells) in the nasal secretions, suggestive of allergy. ASA sensitivity is also the reason for some cases of stubborn, chronic hives that defy treatment. Most people allergic to ASA cross-react and also develop symptoms when taking other NSAIDs, such as indomethacin, naproxen, ibuprofen, meclofenamate, ketoprofen, ketorolac, sulindac or phenylbutazone.

Unfortunately the skin prick and RAST blood tests do not reliably identify those at risk of ASA allergy. The only useful test is a controlled challenge test to check whether ingesting a tiny amount causes symptoms. But this test can be hazardous and must be done by a trained allergist, with emergency resuscitation capability on hand. In general, allergists don't advise these tests unless the benefits of taking the drug outweigh the hazards of allergy testing.

Asthma sufferers are particularly prone to ASA and other NSAID reactions, especially those with the "allergic triad": asthma, sinusitis (chronic nasal inflammation) and nasal polyps. The solution is to stop taking the medications. Symptoms can be relieved with a corticosteroid spray or puffer, and perhaps a bronchodilator to ease airway congestion. Asthma sufferers are often advised to abstain from all ASA and other

NSAIDs. Desensitization with immunotherapy may reduce the sensitivity in those with underlying asthma or nasal polyps, allowing them to take ASA. However, anyone who has had a severe ASA reaction should wear a medical-alert bracelet and carry an emergency epinephrine injector. At the slightest hint of breathing problems as a possible reaction to ASA or another drug, get to the closest hospital emergency unit immediately.

Vaccine Allergies

Immunization has played a key role in improving human health. It involves the injection of vaccines containing small doses of killed (or live but much weakened) infectious agents. The weakened or killed infectious agents trigger the immune system to build antibodies, preparing it to ward off a future attack by the same viruses or bacteria. Apart from safe drinking water and better nutrition, no other medical advance has brought about as great a reduction in illness and death.

Although the benefits of vaccines far outweigh their risks, there is a slight chance of allergic and other reactions. In former times, when the diseases that modern vaccines combat were widespread – and greatly feared – vaccine side-effects were generally accepted as a small price to pay for protection against the ravages of infection. But now that these killer diseases have become rare in North America, vaccine side-effects loom larger in people's minds, and are sometimes exaggerated in the popular press – even to the extent of scaring people off life-saving immunization, or discouraging them from having their children vaccinated.

No vaccine is entirely safe, but most children undergoing routinely scheduled vaccinations feel few adverse effects other than a sore arm or a slight fever for a day or two. But although it's rare, there is an occasional allergic reaction to some vaccines. Such reactions can be triggered by the vaccine itself, by the culture medium (such as chick embryos) in which it's grown or by additives, preservatives or antibiotics used in its preparation. "But," notes one pediatric allergist, "the risk of serious side-effects from vaccination is often blown out of proportion."

The vaccines most likely to trigger allergic reactions are those grown on chick or duck eggs or embryos. Although chicken and duck cultures are being used less and less, some vaccines are still prepared in egg cultures – for instance, measles, mumps, yellow fever and influenza vaccines. These vaccines may therefore trigger allergic reactions, possibly severe, in egg-sensitive people. (Rubella vaccine, formerly grown in duck embryos, is now prepared in human cell cultures.) In general, however, routine MMR (combined measles, mumps and rubella) shots are considered safe even for egg-allergic persons. Many studies show that mumps and measles vaccines can safely be given to most egg-sensitive children. Those allergic to eggs should be skin-tested before receiving yellow-fever vaccine, as it may contain more egg protein. And

The debate over MMR

There has been some debate in both the U.S. and Canada about the need for, and feasibility of, pretesting egg-allergic people before administering the MMR (measles, mumps and rubella) vaccine. A recent Ontario study on measles reimmunization found an unexpectedly high rate of allergy-type reactions – about 7 per 100,000 vaccinations, and 2 suspected cases of anaphylaxis. The researchers conducting this survey suggest that the unusually high rate may be partly due to the inclusion of skin blotchiness as a symptom; blotches arising from anxiety may have been mislabeled as allergy-like reactions. A U.S. study of college students in a recent measles revaccination campaign found far lower rates of allergy-type reactions.

MMR vaccines may also contain traces of the antibiotic neomycin, and people sensitive to it may have a severe reaction. It's wise to tell the administering doctor or nurse about a possible allergic response before being immunized.

anyone known to be allergic to eggs should not have a flu shot until skin testing has been done and such immunization is considered safe.

Healthcare providers giving vaccines watch for the possibility of anaphylaxis, are familiar with its symptoms and should be ready to administer resuscitation. Recipients are usually monitored for at least 15 minutes after vaccination. Canadian statistics show an annual rate of seven to ten cases of suspected vaccine-related allergic reaction per 100,000 doses of all vaccine injected. In 1996 the Canadian Society of Allergy and Clinical Immunology issued guidelines for managing vaccine-induced anaphylaxis, and parallel U.S. guidelines have also been developed.

FIFTEEN

Summing It Up

Over the last few decades, scientists have made considerable strides in understanding the underpinnings of allergic reactions and refining treatments. New medications and therapies are constantly being developed. For example, we already have the first mediator blockers on the market; and vaccines that block IgE production and may prevent the allergic response by turning off the mast cells' mediator release are in the early testing phase. So the future looks bright for better allergy control.

Even today, more than 90 percent of those with hay fever and allergic rhinitis can effectively control their symptoms and keep down the discomfort, without troublesome side-effects; eye symptoms are also manageable, using drops safe for the eyes. Many asthma sufferers can now manage their disease effectively with the new array of anti-inflammatory medications. But much remains to be done in educating asthmatics and their caregivers about the disease, and helping all asthmatics develop an action plan for worsening symptoms – alerting them to the need to increase medication, or to go to the nearest emergency unit for help.

Controlling and Living with Allergies

In most people, allergy symptoms are unpleasant and aggravating but not life-endangering. They can generally be adequately treated with over-the-counter antihistamines and other nonprescription medications. People with more severe allergies, or whose symptoms don't respond to over-the-counter remedies, may require ongoing care by a physician.

In many cases, especially when there is an inherited predisposition to atopy, "cure" is impossible and people must learn to live with their allergies. This can be difficult at first, and some people resent the changes in lifestyle imposed by their allergic disorder, especially a severe one such as chronic hives or asthma. A serious allergy problem can dramatically undermine self-perception, and some people get depressed to the point of requiring antidepressant therapy. Others deal with the allergy by denying its existence, and even reject or neglect to follow the suggested treatment. But once people accept and adapt to having a chronic disorder – one that's likely to last a lifetime – they have overcome the main hurdle in managing it and getting on with their lives.

The best bet is to aim for "control" – keeping the discomfort (and possible danger) at bay. This is eminently achievable in most cases, with appropriate medical advice. The key is to remove or avoid the offending allergens if possible, use medications wisely and seek specialized help when needed. The host of new medications now available, properly prescribed and properly used, allow many allergy sufferers to lead normal lives.

Immunotherapy, one of the oldest therapies for allergy, is being refined, and there are now clear guidelines for its use. Purified allergen extracts have been developed and studies have identified those most likely to benefit from allergy shots, with minimal risk. For some people, immunotherapy now ranks as an allergy "cure."

However, not all allergy treatment is a success story. Food allergy, for example, is still managed more or less as it was in the time of Hippocrates: "If it makes you sick, don't eat it." No new drugs or therapies are yet on the horizon for food allergy. Severe eczema, chronic hives and contact dermatitis remain major problems for many thousands of sufferers.

One stumbling block is the scarcity of accurate statistics. It's hard to know, for example, the extent to which peanut allergy is increasing, because there are no accurate statistics on its incidence in the first place, or on the number of North Americans who die every year from peanut or any other kind of allergy. Throughout this book we have used the most reliable numbers available, but many of them are merely "best guesses."

Allergy awareness is on the rise these days, and allergy associations have sprung up with offices across the continent to increase public education, disseminate information and help those living with allergies. Publicity and education about allergies and the potential dangers of severe reactions have increased public awareness of the problems and needs of allergic people – for instance, in regard to home design, and building and furnishing materials. In some U.S. and Canadian cities, experimental "allergy-free" homes are being constructed as prototypes of less allergy-provoking environments to live in.

Food labels are becoming more accurate but many still don't clearly list all ingredients. Allergy associations are publishing guidelines for protecting severely food-allergic children in schools; some restaurants now offer "allergy-free" menus. There are also new guidelines for protecting latex-sensitive healthcare workers.

Attempts to forestall or minimize allergic reactions by avoidance tactics can be time-consuming, tiring and expensive. Allergy experts have many tips on what's worthwhile and what isn't, as well as information about what unconventional or unproven methods are likely to work. Some people build special environmentally controlled houses to rid themselves of their allergic discomfort. How much is too much is a matter of opinion. As one man complained, his children "could no longer behave like children," as his wife, who was allergic to "everything *and* the kitchen sink, " kept the house so obsessively clean that the children led very restricted lives. People with allergies can apply to allergy and asthma associations for consumer information on allergy-free products, home-cleaning strategies and general information about their disease (see the resource section).

A confusing diversity of anti-allergy medications, in different forms and varied dispensers, is flooding the market, and it's best to consult a physician about which ones suit your particular allergic situation. It's crucial to understand the action

---

Expert tips on adjusting to an allergic disorder

- Communicate the problem to those close to you, and to your care-givers, to gain support and aid in achieving control.
- Ask physicians to clearly explain the treatment prescribed and why it's suggested. If you don't understand, ask for a repeat explanation.
- Discuss your concerns with caregivers.
- Always have your doctor's phone number handy, in case of need.
- If cigarette smoke, perfumes or other irritants aggravate your allergy, speak out!
- If your condition seems to worsen, or becomes suddenly severe, tell those close to you and call for medical help; don't deny its severity or try to "tough it out."
- If you're an asthma sufferer, don't be overcomplacent. Understand your disease, and get specialized medical advice in managing it.

of any medication taken, know how it should be used (especially for inhaled medications), the right dosage and timing, and any side-effects to watch for. It's also necessary to ask about possible interactions with other drugs you take, as some combinations cause ill effects, or the drugs may cancel each other out.

In cases of really severe allergy – particularly asthma – the balance of precaution and normal life is a personal matter. One rational strategy for weighing the risks and benefits of allergy control is to start with the cheapest, simplest and most conservative measures, and those least disruptive to yourself and your family, and see how well they work, before moving on to more expensive or drastic measures.

For example, one mother whose seven-year-old has a life-threatening anaphylactic peanut allergy is philosophical about it: "Oh well, what can we do? We can't protect him all his life. We give him an EpiPen, teach him when and how to use it and let him get on with things. We don't want to be over-protective and overemotional. After all, he's more likely to get killed by a car than to die of a peanut, and I'm not always in a lather about cars." This approach of downplaying even a life-threatening allergy may seem rational and calm to some, but heartless and blasé – even foolhardy – to others. Much depends on the maturity and the personalities of the people involved.

I hope this book has given you enough evidence-based information to make sensible decisions in managing your allergy. Remember that many new solutions to allergies are being studied, and new products are constantly coming onto the market. For more information about allergies, allergy associations and anti-allergy products, please see the resource section at the end of this book.

Glossary

Action-plan (for asthma): a plan devised by an asthmatic and his/her medical caregivers, to be put into action at predetermined signs of deteriorating breathing ability.

Acute (of a disease or disorder): having a sudden onset and a short, sometimes severe course.

Add-on (accessory) devices: tubes or small containers (also called "spacers") added to metered-dose inhalers, allowing the aerosolized medication to be sprayed into the airways with less meticulous timing.

Adrenalin: a hormone naturally produced by the body's adrenal gland (especially in times of fear or stress) that increases the heart rate and constricts blood vessels. *See also* **Epinephrine.**

Adrenergic: activated by, characteristic of or secreting adrenalin (epinephrine), or

substances with similar biological activity.

Aerosol: medication supplied as a fine mist.

Airway obstruction: a narrowing, clogging or blocking of the breathing passages.

Allergen: any substance – usually a protein – that creates allergic sensitization and induces an immunological reaction. *See also* **Antigen.**

Allergic reaction: immune-system overreaction provoked by contact with normally harmless substances such as pollen, molds, foods or cosmetics.

Allergic rhinitis: an IgE-mediated allergic reaction involving inflammation of the nasal membranes, caused by an inhaled allergen such as pollen, animal debris or mold.

Allergist: a physician with specialized training in the body's immune system, the science of immunology and allergy-related disorders.

Allergy: an inappropriate or overly strong response by the body's immune system to normally innocuous substances, resulting in identifiable (sometimes severe) symptoms.

Alveoli: air sacs at the ends of the lung's bronchioles, where oxygen is absorbed into the bloodstream.

Anaphylactic reaction: a severe allergic response with rapid changes in many systems of the body, including widespread hives, swelling, airway blockage, breathing difficulty, blood-vessel expansion and "leakiness" – causing a sudden drop in blood pressure – which may lead to shock, collapse, heart stoppage and even death.

Anaphylaxis: an immediate, rapid, severe (possibly life-threatening) reaction involving many body systems at once.

Angioedema: swelling of the skin's deeper layers.

Antibodies: special protein molecules (made by white blood cells) that bind to foreign particles (antigens) when they enter the body; the "allergy antibody," immunoglobulin E (IgE), triggers allergic symptoms.

Anticholinergic agent: a type of bronchodilating (airway-widening) agent used as an add-on medication for asthma.

Antigen: any foreign protein or other agent that, when introduced into the body, stimulates the production of antibodies. (Allergens are one type of antigen.)

Antihistamine: a drug that relieves some allergy symptoms by blocking the action of histamine.

Anti-inflammatory medication: a substance that reduces inflammatory swelling and discomfort.

ASA (acetylsalicylic acid): a painkiller, fever reducer and anti-inflammatory agent used as an ingredient in many products – e.g., in headache remedies and some decongestants. Also called "aspirin" in the U.S. (In Canada "Aspirin" is a brand name for ASA.)

Asthma: a disorder in which the airways become inflamed, constricted and blocked by mucus. Symptoms are wheezing, coughing and shortness of breath.

Atopic: subject to **Atopy**.

Atopic dermatitis: *see* **Eczema**.

Atopy: an inherited tendency to develop allergic disorders, with an oversensitive immune system that produces above-average amounts of IgE antibody.

Autonomic: involuntary or automatic – often applied to the part of the nervous system that acts without our conscious knowledge or command.

Basophil: type of white blood cell in bloodstream that releases chemical mediators during an allergic reaction.

B-cells: white blood cells, derived from bone marrow, that produce IgE antibodies – also called "B-lymphocytes."

Beta agonist: a drug that stimulates the beta receptors – e.g., in lung tissue, expanding the airways to ease breathing.

Beta blockers: drugs to reduce blood pressure.

Beta receptor: the site in certain body tissues that responds to stimulation by specific drugs and related substances.

B-lymphocytes: *see* **B-cells.**

Bronchi: large air passages leading from the trachea to the lungs.

Bronchial hyperactivity: extra-sensitive or "twitchy" reaction of the airways to stimuli such as cold air – linked to asthma.

Bronchial tubes: tubes through which air passes from the nose and mouth into the lungs, and back out again.

Bronchioles: tiny, branching extensions of the bronchi inside the lungs.

Bronchitis: inflammation of the bronchi, arising from irritation or a viral or bacterial infection.

Bronchodilators: inhaled medications that relax smooth muscle and widen constricted air passages, making it easier for people with blocked airways to breathe.

Bronchospasm: contraction of the muscles encircling the airways, narrowing the breathing passages.

Challenge testing: a method of testing for food (or other) allergies in which the person is exposed to a tiny amount of the substance and symptoms are observed. In an "open" challenge, the person knows which substance is being tried; in a "blind" challenge, the presence or absence of the suspected allergen is disguised.

Chronic: tending to occur regularly over a long period.

Conjunctivitis: inflammation of the conjunctiva – the membranes lining the eyelid – with swelling, itching, redness and watering of the eye.

Contact dermatitis: a skin rash triggered by touching or rubbing a material or chemical.

Corticosteroids: natural or synthetic hormones used as anti-inflammatory agents in the treatment of allergic reactions and asthma.

Cytokines: chemical messengers secreted by lymphocytes (e.g., by TH2-helper cells) that cause other cells to react (e.g., cause B-cells to produce and release IgE antibodies).

Dander: tiny scales of animal skin and hair mixed with dried saliva.

Decongestant: a medication that reduces nasal congestion.

Degranulate: release mediator chemicals from granules of mast cells or basophils in response to an allergen invasion and IgE-antibody activity.

Desensitization: *see* **Immunotherapy.**

Dilate: expand.

Dust mite: a tiny insect that lives on dead skin scales in house dust. Its feces cause allergies.

Eczema: an itchy, noncontagious skin condition that can be flaky or wet and weepy. Eczema is sometimes due to an allergy (atopic eczema), but not always.

Emphysema: a chronic, irreversible lung disease characterized by a breakdown of the walls of the lungs' alveoli.

Eosinophil: a white blood cell that is part of the body's immune defenses; a collection of eosinophils at an attack site can cause an inflammatory reaction (as in an asthma attack). Elevated numbers indicate an allergic reaction.

Epinephrine: adrenalin (often synthetic) taken by injection for the treatment of severe allergic reactions or anaphylaxis. The terms "epinephrine," "adrenalin" and "adrenaline" are often used interchangeably.

Forced expired volume (FEV): the maximum volume of air that a person can forcibly breathe out of the lungs in a certain time (usually one second), after taking in a full breath.

Fungal: pertaining to or caused by fungus.

Fungus: organisms such as yeast, mushrooms and molds.

Hapten: a molecule in the body that may attach to small allergens.

Hay fever: seasonal allergic rhinitis, which causes nasal discomfort, itching, swelling, congestion and a clear discharge – usually triggered by pollens from trees, grasses or weeds.

HEPA filters: high-efficiency particulate air filters for air-conditioning and heating units, to curb indoor allergen levels.

Histamine: an organic chemical or "mediator" released by mast cells and basophils in an allergic reaction, responsible for much of the swelling, itching and allergic discomfort.

Hives (urticaria): itchy skin weals with white, raised areas surrounded by redness. Can look like a cluster of mosquito bites, or appear as large welts.

Hypersensitivity: overreaction to normally harmless stimuli or substances.

Hypoallergenic: containing lower than usual amounts of allergen – but not necessarily allergen-free.

IgE antibody: an antibody normally made in small amounts, but manufactured inappropriately by allergy-prone people. IgE antibodies attach to mast cells and basophils and trigger the mediator release that produces allergic symptoms.

IgE-mediated: occurring because of IgE-antibody activity.

Immune system: a collection of cells and chemicals in the body that defends it against attack or invasion by foreign materials such as viruses, bacteria, fungi, parasites and poisons.

Immunoglobulin: protein molecules that act as antibodies and are part of the body's immune defenses. There are different types (immunoglobulin A, G, E and so on). Immunoglobulin E (IgE) is the allergy antibody.

Immunotherapy: a series of injections of allergen extracts – commonly referred to as "allergy shots" or "desensitization" – aimed at abolishing or dampening the reaction to specific allergens.

Inflammation: tissue swelling, redness, heat and pain – the result of fluid leaking out of blood vessels into the surrounding area.

Inhalant allergens: allergens that enter the body through the nose, such as dust, pollen, animal dander and molds.

Inhaler: a device to provide medications inhaled into the lungs as aerosolized drops or powder.

Irritant: anything that irritates or worsens symptoms. Cold air can act as an irritant that sets off an asthma attack; cosmetics can irritate the skin.

Late-phase: the stage of symptoms that occurs several hours after exposure to an allergen, as opposed to immediate allergic responses.

Leukocytes: white blood cells.

Leukotrienes: biologically active compounds, released by mast cells and basophils, that act as mediators in an allergic response, contracting smooth muscle: e.g., constricting the airways.

Lymphocytes: specialized white blood cells that participate in immune and allergic responses; part of the body's defense system.

Macrophages: large white blood cells that act as "scavengers," engulfing microorganisms and antigens.

Mast cells: cells in the mucous membranes that release chemicals called mediators (such as histamine, bradykinin, leukotriene), which cause the symptoms typical of allergic reactions.

Mediators: potent chemicals released from basophils and mast cells, responsible for the symptoms of allergic disease.

Metered-dose inhaler (MDI): a small, sometimes pressurized canister that dispenses aerosol medications, often used for asthma.

Mucosal tissue: soft layers of lining tissue just below the skin's surface, and in the respiratory tract and digestive tract, containing many mast cells.

Mucous membrane: *see* **Mucosal tissue.**

Mucus: phlegm, or slimy discharge from mucosal tissue.

Nebulizer: a device requiring a power source and compressor to deliver a mist of aerosolized medication, usually through a mask; used in some asthma cases.

NSAIDs: Nonsteroidal anti-inflammatory drugs.

Peak flow meter: a hand-held device with a mouthpiece and spring gauge to measure the force with which someone can expel air from the lungs, to determine the extent of obstruction.

Pulmonary: having to do with the lungs.

Radioallergosorbent test (RAST): a blood test that measures the level of IgE antibodies to a particular allergen.

Respiratory tract: the passages of the breathing apparatus, including mouth, nose, throat, windpipe, bronchi and lungs.

Rhinitis: inflammation of the mucous membranes lining the nose, with itching, swelling, congestion and a clear discharge.

Rhinoconjunctivitis: inflammation, redness, itching, watering and discharge in both nose and eyes.

Seasonal allergic rhinitis: *see* **Hay fever.**

Sensitization: allergic sensitivity caused by exposure to a specific allergen, leading to a reaction on re-exposure.

Serum sickness: a complex reaction (often to drugs) with a rash, fever, swelling of the face, eyelids or lips, puffiness in the hands and feet, and joint pain.

Skin prick test: an allergy test that involves pricking or scratching the skin on parts of the back or arms, applying a drop of allergen-containing solution and observing the reaction. A reddened spot indicates a positive reaction.

Spacers: assorted tubes or chambers attached to

pressurized metered-dose inhalers to ease medication delivery.

Spirometer: an instrument that measures the flow of air in and out of the lungs.

Sputum: secretion from the lower passages of the lungs, expelled by coughing.

Stimulus: any agent, act, event or influence that produces functional changes in the body.

Sulfites: a group of food additives (e.g., metabisulfites) that can cause allergies or exacerbate asthma.

Systemic: a reaction that spreads to affect many body systems at once, usually involving the blood circulation and breathing system.

T-cells: white blood cells that are processed in the thymus gland, and participate in cell-mediated immune-system responses.

T-helper cells: a type of lymphocyte (white blood cell) involved in the body's immune defenses.

TH1-helper cells: specific lymphocytes that primarily make interferon, an anti-viral agent.

TH2-helper cells: specific lymphocytes that secrete cytokines (chemical messengers) that incite B-lymphocytes to make IgE antibodies.

Tolerance: the ability to encounter a certain amount of allergen or irritant without reacting adversely.

Topical: (of a medication or other substance) – applied to a surface area or specific site, such as the skin or the nasal passages.

Total allergy syndrome ("20th-century disease"): a term now largely replaced by "multiple chemical sensitivity," to denote sensitivity – but *not* proven allergy – to multiple environmental agents.

Trachea: the windpipe – extending from the larynx to the two bronchi.

Twentieth-century disease: *see* **Total allergy syndrome.**

Type 1 allergic reaction: immediate or fast-onset allergic reaction that involves IgE-antibodies.

Urticaria: *see* **Hives.**

Vasoactive: affecting the vascular (blood-vessel) system.

Vasoconstrictor: an agent or medication that constricts the blood vessels.

Wheezing: a whistling sound when someone breathes out through narrowed or inflamed bronchial tubes; a frequent sign of asthma.

Further Resources

Organizations

Canada

Allergy, Asthma and
Immunology Society of Ontario
2 Demaris Avenue
Downsview, ON M3N 1M1
(416) 633-2215
Fax: (416) 633-3108

Allergy/Asthma Information
Association
30 Eglinton Avenue W.
Suite 750
Mississauga, ON L5R 3E7
(905) 712-2242

Allergy and Environmental
Health Association
513 Quiet Place
Waterloo, ON N2L 5L6
(519) 885-2803

Anaphylaxis Foundation
of Canada
3080 Yonge Street, Suite 2054
Toronto, ON M4N 3N1

Anaphylaxis Network
133 The West Mall, Unit 9
Etobicoke, ON M9C 1C2
(416) 785-4684

Asthma Society of Canada
130 Bridgeland Avenue, Suite 425
Toronto, ON M6A 1Z4
(416) 787-4050

Canadian Lung Association
1900 City Park Drive, Suite 508
Blair Business Park
Gloucester, ON K1J 1A3
(613) 747-6776
Fax: (613) 747-7430

Canadian Society of Allergy and
Clinical Immunology
774 Echo Drive
Ottawa, ON K2P 5N8
(613) 730-6272
1-800-668-3740 ext. 272

C.A.N.DO (Movement
for Clean Air)
Ontario Lung Association
365 Bloor Street E., Suite 601
Toronto, ON M4W 3L9
(416) 922-9440

Dietitians of Canada
480 University Avenue
Suite 601
Toronto, ON M5G 1V2
(416) 596-0857

International Asthma Council
195 Parkview Hill Crescent
Toronto, ON M4B 1S2
(416) 750-7961

Medic Alert Foundation Inc.
250 Ferrand Drive
Toronto, ON M3C 2T9
(416) 696-0267

U.S.A.

Allergy and Asthma Network/
Mothers of Asthmatics
3554 Chain Bridge Road, #200
Fairfax, VA 22030-2709
(703) 385-4403

Allergy-Free Inc.
1502 Pine Drive
Dickinson, TX 77539
(713) 337-3764
Toll-free: 1-800-ALLERGY
Fax: (713) 337-5897

American Academy of Allergy,
Asthma & Immunology
611 East Wells Street
Milwaukee, WI 53202
(414) 272-6071

American Allergy Association
P.O. Box 7273
Menlo Park, CA 94926
(415) 322-1663

American College of Allergy,
Asthma and Immunology
85 W. Algonquin Road
Suite 550
Arlington Heights, IL 60005
(847) 427-1200

American Dietetic Association
216 West Jackson Blvd.
Chicago IL 60606-6995
(312) 899-4855

American Lung Association
1740 Broadway
New York, NY 10019-4374
(212) 315-8700

Asthma and Allergy
Foundation of America
1125 15th Street NW
Suite 502
Washington, DC 20005
(202) 466-7643

Asthma Care Association
of America
P.O. Box 568
Spring Valley Road
Ossining, NY 10362
(212) 288-5416

Food Allergy Network
10400 Eaton Place, Suite 107
Fairfax, VA 22030-2208
(703) 691-3179

Medic Alert Foundation
International
2424 Colorado Avenue
Turlock, CA 95382
1-800-432-5378

National Asthma Education &
Prevention Project
National Heart, Lung and Blood
Institute
31 Center Drive, MSC 2480
Bethesda, MD 20892-2480
(301) 496-4236

Books and Journals

Allergies: The Complete Guide to Diagnosis, Treatment, and Daily Management. 1992. Consumer Reports.

Allergy Asthma Quarterly. Allergy/Asthma Information Association, Canada (see address above).

Allergy Encyclopedia. 1991. Asthma and Allergy Foundation of America.

Bachman, J. 1992. *Keys to Dealing with Childhood Allergy.* Barron.

Beaudette, Thérèse. 1991. *Adverse Reactions to Foods.* American Dietetic Association.

Boutin, H., and L. Boulet. 1995. *Understand and Control Your Asthma.* McGill-Queen's University Press.

Dobler, M.L. *Food Allergies.* 1991. American Dietetic Association.

Donaldson, John. 1994. *Living with Asthma and Hay Fever.* Penguin.

Newhouse, M., and P. Barnes. 1991. *Conquering Asthma.* Book Art Inc.

Novick, N.L. 1994. *You Can Do Something about Your Allergies.* Macmillan/Bantam.

Priorities (publications and catalog of anti-allergy products). Available from 70 Walnut Street, Wellesley, MA 02181, U.S.A. Telephone (617) 239-8123 or 1-800-553-5398; fax (617) 239-7559; http://www.priorities.com

Sussman, G., and M. Gold. 1996. *Guidelines for the Management of Latex Allergies.* CHA Press, Ottawa.

Tames, P. 1993. *The Asthma Handbook.* Canadian Lung Association (see address above).

Zimmerman, B., M. Gold, S. Lavi and S. Feanny. Revised 1996. *Canadian Allergy and Asthma Handbook.* Random House, Canada.

Index